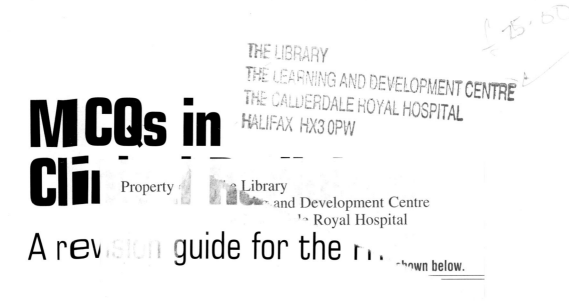

MCQs in
Clinical Radiology

A revision guide for the m...

JRG Bell, NH Davies, N Jeyadevan, DM Koh

This book was conceived when we were Specialist Registrars
at the Chelsea and Westminster Hospital, London, UK.

Published by the Remedica Group

Remedica Publishing, 32–38 Osnaburgh Street, London, NW1 3ND, UK
Remedica Inc, Tri-State International Center, Building 25, Suite 150, Lincolnshire, IL 60069, USA

E-mail: books@remedica.com
www.remedica.com

Publisher: Andrew Ward
In-house editors: Thomas Moberly and Helen James

ISBN 1 901346 2 69
British Library Cataloguing-in-Publication Data
A catalogue record for this book is available from the British Library

MCQs in Clinical Radiology

A revision guide for the FRCR

JRG Bell, BSc, MRCP, FRCR
Consultant Radiologist
Royal Free Hospital, London, UK

NH Davies, FRCS, FRCR
Consultant Interventional Radiologist
Royal Free Hospital, London, UK

N Jeyadevan, MRCP, FRCR
Consultant Radiologist
Mayday Hospital, London, UK

DM Koh, MRCP, FRCR
Senior Lecturer and Honorary Consultant
Royal Marsden Hospital, Surrey, UK

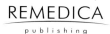

REMEDICA
publishing

LONDON • CHICAGO

Preface

The idea of writing a new multiple choice question (MCQ) book came soon after some of us completed the Fellow of the Royal College of Radiologists (FRCR) examinations. It was apparent that the FRCR MCQ papers tested knowledge and understanding beyond the scope of standard radiology textbooks. Although there are already a number of existing radiology MCQ books on the market, many of these place a lesser emphasis on computed tomography (CT) and magnetic resonance imaging (MRI), which have become the cornerstones in many aspects of modern radiology. In addition, the earlier books did not embrace the newer developments in ultrasonography, nuclear medicine and positron emission tomography (PET) imaging, which have emerged in the last few years.

In setting the MCQs, we have tried to retain a mixture of the 'old' and the 'new', with emphasis on the latter, especially with regards to CT and MRI. We have spent considerable time trawling through specialist textbooks and recent journal review articles to tease out the state-of-the-art imaging and current knowledge. These are translated into MCQs to test the initiated and inform those who are unaware. The answers to each question are expanded to provide a summary of the key facts of the diseases under review. We hope this will provide candidates with the opportunity to consolidate their knowledge, by focusing on traditional examination 'favourites', whilst also presenting the many new aspects of clinical imaging.

The chapters in this book are organised by subspeciality and organ systems instead of by examination format for two reasons. Firstly, this allows candidates to utilise this book during revision of a particular subspeciality, rather than at the end of their study. Areas of weakness identified in attempting the MCQs can be promptly addressed by further reading into the relevant areas. Secondly, with the introduction of the new modular format for the FRCR, learning and revising by subspeciality and organ system is now more important than ever.

The field of radiology is expanding at a phenomenal rate. Our thoughts are with the candidates who have the unenviable task of assimilating this large body of information. We can only wish them every success in their examinations.

JRG Bell
NH Davies
N Jeyadevan
DM Koh

Foreword

It is generally believed by candidates for the multiple-choice component of the final FRCR exam that the questions undergo rapid gestation from casual suggestions proposed by the examiners over a fine dinner! After 5 years experience as one such examiner, I am able to assert that nothing is further from the truth. Hundreds of questions begin their life in centres all around the UK from whence they are submitted by chairmen of regional panels. Their submitted questions are then subjected to detailed examination by a small group of examiners after which many are determined still-born. Those few that progress suffer further detailed examination from the full Examining Board over a 2-day sojourn in the basement of the Royal College of Radiologists. Only then do a few reach maturity to be included in the Final Examination.

For a quartet of young radiologists to consider the creation of their own collection of multiple choice questions is both ambitious and challenging. I am pleased to report that none had any individual experience of the Part IIa FRCR beyond a single sitting, and to produce such a high quality monograph in so short a time is truly an outstanding achievement.

Diagnostic imaging is in constant evolution, and the rate of change has been truly phenomenal over the past ten to fifteen years. It is a necessary requirement, therefore, that examinations change in accordance with change in clinical practice, and this contemporary book responds to that by including many questions pertinent to modern radiological practice as well as the current radiology curriculum.

Fear of the unknown dominates the experience of most patients embarking on an episode in the healthcare system today. A not dissimilar fear of the unknown is demonstrated by virtually every candidate approaching the MCQ. I have no doubt that completion of the questions in this text will prove both factually and emotionally educational by providing an accurate and very relevant insight into the characteristics of the examination.

I am full of admiration for the energy of the authors, and am delighted to be able to commend this collection of multiple choice questions to every training radiologist.

Dr. Michael King
Consultant Radiologist, Royal Marsden Hospital, London

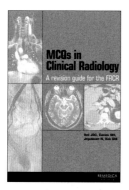

Contents

Chapter 1

Thoracic radiology

1   **When a solitary pulmonary nodule is seen on computed tomography (CT), which of the following radiological features suggest it is benign?**
    a) Air bronchograms within the nodule
    b) Amorphous calcification within the nodule
    c) CT attenuation of −10 Hounsfield units (HU)
    d) Lobulated outline of the nodule
    e) Enhancement of the nodule by less than 15 HU following intravenous contrast

2   **In the staging of nonsmall cell carcinoma of the lung, which of the following are true?**
    a) Ipsilateral hilar lymph node involvement is a contraindication to surgery
    b) Malignant effusion contraindicates curative resection
    c) Involvement of the pericardium indicates unresectability
    d) Rib invasion is a contraindication to surgery
    e) Tumour involvement of the main pulmonary veins indicates T4 disease

3   **In using magnetic resonance imaging (MRI) to stage nonsmall cell carcinoma of the lung, which of the following are true?**
    a) Lymph node metastases in the aorto-pulmonary window are better evaluated with CT than MRI
    b) T2-weighted images are most useful in the assessment of chest wall invasion
    c) MRI is the best modality to assess superior sulcus tumours
    d) CT is superior to MRI in the assessment of mediastinal invasion
    e) MRI signal characteristics allow discrimination between normal and infiltrated lymph nodes

4   **Which of the following are causes of superior vena cava obstruction (SVCO)?**
    a) Lymphoma
    b) Central venous line
    c) Aortic aneurysm
    d) Constrictive pericarditis
    e) Histoplasmosis

5   **Which of the following are true regarding bronchoalveolar carcinoma?**
    a) There is an increased incidence in patients with systemic sclerosis
    b) Spontaneous radiographic improvement may occur
    c) Small cystic lucent areas are frequently seen on CT
    d) Pleural effusions are rare
    e) A negative positron emission tomography (PET) scan excludes the diagnosis

6   **Which of the following are true regarding bronchial carcinoid tumours?**
    a) The chest radiograph is normal in most cases at presentation
    b) A solitary nodule in the lung periphery is the most common radiographic finding
    c) It is a cause of Cushing's syndrome
    d) It results in carcinoid syndrome in 50% of cases
    e) An atypical carcinoid frequently metastasises to the hilar lymph nodes

7   Which of the following are true regarding squamous cell carcinoma of the lung?
a)   It presents with a peripheral mass in 30%–40% of cases
b)   It is a recognised cause of antidiuretic hormone (ADH) secretion
c)   It cavitates in 20% of cases
d)   It metastasises more frequently than small-cell lung carcinoma
e)   It is the most common histological type in Pancoast tumour

8   Which of the following statements regarding pulmonary neoplasms are true?
a)   Pulmonary hamartomas show popcorn calcifications on radiography in 60% of cases
b)   There is an association of pulmonary chondromas with adrenal paragangliomas
c)   Primary pulmonary lymphoma is usually Hodgkin's type
d)   A mass with an attenuation value of 200 HU on CT is usually benign
e)   Multiple calcified nodules are a feature of pulmonary amyloidosis

9   Which of the following are true regarding intrathoracic Hodgkin's lymphoma?
a)   Lymphadenopathy is typically bilateral and symmetrical
b)   Posterior mediastinal lymph nodes are commonly involved
c)   Pulmonary involvement is usually perihilar
d)   Pleural effusion is frequently accompanied by mediastinal lymphadenopathy
e) ^{67}Gallium radionuclide scan is useful to monitor response to treatment

10 Which of the following are true regarding benign pleural fibroma?
a)   It has an association with asbestosis
b)   It is a cause of hypertrophic osteoarthropathy
c)   It is a cause of hyperglycaemia
d)   Calcification is common
e)   Pedunculation is common

11 Which of the following are true regarding malignant mesothelioma?
a)   Selective involvement of the parietal pleura is typical
b)   Circumferential pleural thickening is typical
c)   It is a cause of hypertrophic osteoarthropathy
d)   Pleural effusions are common
e)   Chest wall invasion occurs in 12% of cases at presentation

12 Which of the following are causes of nodular pleural masses?
a)   Splenosis
b)   Malignant thymoma
c)   Lymphoma
d)   Metastatic ovarian carcinoma
e)   Asbestosis

13 Which of the following are true regarding pulmonary metastases?
a)   Thin-walled cysts are a feature of treated metastatic transitional cell carcinoma
b)   Miliary metastases commonly result from breast carcinoma
c)   Endobronchial metastases occur with renal cell carcinoma
d)   Lymphangitis carcinomatosa may result from prostatic carcinoma
e)   Calcified metastases are commonly seen with colonic carcinoma

14 **Which of the following are true regarding thymoma?**
   a) More than 60% of patients with thymoma have myasthenia gravis
   b) It has an association with hypogammaglobulinaemia
   c) Calcification is commonly seen on CT
   d) Haematogenous metastases occur frequently with malignant thymoma
   e) It is more common in females

15 **Which of the following are true regarding Castleman's disease?**
   a) It typically occurs in the elderly
   b) CT demonstrates nodal mass with uniform enhancement following intravenous contrast
   c) Nodal calcification is a feature
   d) Lymph nodes frequently cavitate
   e) It may involve lymph nodes in the retroperitoneum

16 **Which of the following are true regarding *Mycobacterium tuberculosis* infection?**
   a) Miliary tuberculosis heals with small focal calcifications
   b) It results in broncholithiasis
   c) Pleural effusions are more common in postprimary disease
   d) CT is more useful than bronchoscopy in the assessment of post-tuberculous bronchial strictures
   e) Branching y or v densities ('tree-in-bud') on high resolution CT indicates active infection

17 **Which of the following are true regarding round pneumonia?**
   a) It occurs most commonly in the second and third decades of life
   b) It is more common in the upper lobes
   c) It is most commonly associated with *Klebsiella* infection
   d) It frequently progresses to cavitation
   e) It is a feature of Q-fever infection

18 **Which of the following are true regarding pulmonary infections?**
   a) Consolidation due to viral pneumonia frequently cavitates
   b) Pulmonary infarction may result from Klebsiella pneumonia
   c) Pleural effusions are common with *Chlamydia pneumoniae* infection
   d) Lymphadenopathy is rarely seen in pertussis
   e) Obliterative bronchiolitis occurs in *Mycoplasma* infection

19 **Which of the following are causes of hilar lymph node calcifications?**
   a) Amyloidosis
   b) *Pneumocystis carinii* infection
   c) Berylliosis
   d) Asbestosis
   e) Coal miners' pneumoconiosis

20 **Which of the following are true regarding silicosis?**
   a) It predominantly affects the lower lobes in acute silicoproteinosis
   b) It mimics sarcoidosis on high resolution computed tomography (HRCT)
   c) Emphysema is associated with the development of progressive massive fibrosis
   d) It is a more frequent cause of nodal egg-shell calcification on radiograph than coal miner's pneumoconiosis
   e) Impairment of the lung function test correlates best with the profusion of nodules

21 Which of the following are true regarding asbestos-related diseases?
a) Asbestos-related pleural plaques frequently spare the mediastinal surface
b) Asbestos-related pleural plaques do not extend into interlobular fissures
c) Isolated pleural effusion is a feature
d) Subpleural lower lobe fibrosis is typical of asbestosis
e) Asbestosis is associated with calcified pleural plaques in 20% of cases

22 When a mass-like lesion is seen on CT, which of the following findings support the diagnosis of rounded atelectasis?
a) An anteromedial location of the mass
b) An acute angle with the pleural margins
c) Adjacent pleural thickening
d) Localised crowding of the pulmonary vasculature
e) Absence of enhancement following intravenous contrast

23 Which of the following are true regarding the effects of radiation on the lungs?
a) The severity of the lung changes is related to the fractionation of the radiation dose
b) Acute radiation change usually occurs within 1 month of treatment
c) Pleural effusion usually occurs as a late sequela to radiotherapy
d) Radiation fibrosis is established within 6 months of radiotherapy
e) Pulmonary oligaemia is a feature of the post-irradiated lung

24 Which of the following are true regarding usual interstitial pneumonitis (UIP)?
a) It is more common in females than males
b) It is the most common cause of cryptogenic fibrosing alveolitis
c) It occurs most frequently in the sixth decade of life
d) Areas of ground glass attenuation on HRCT in the absence of parenchymal distortion indicate reversibility
e) A confident diagnosis cannot be made on HRCT without lung biopsy

25 Which of the following are true regarding rheumatoid arthritis with lung involvement?
a) Isolated pleural effusions are more common in men
b) Rheumatoid nodules usually predate the onset of arthritis
c) Rheumatoid nodules have a predilection for the lower lobes
d) There is an increased incidence of bronchiectasis
e) Mosaic lung attenuation is a feature

26 Which of the following are true regarding systemic lupus erythematosus (SLE)?
a) Pleural effusions are common
b) There is an increased incidence of venous thrombosis
c) There is an increased incidence of diaphragmatic dysfunction
d) Respiratory failure from interstitial fibrosis is the most common cause of death
e) Bilateral air-space shadowing is most commonly due to pulmonary haemorrhage

27 **Which of the following statements are true?**
   a) Aspiration pneumonia is common in patients with polymyositis
   b) Pleural effusions are commonly seen in systemic sclerosis
   c) There is a higher incidence of lymphocytic interstitial pneumonia in patients with Sjögren's syndrome
   d) Relapsing polychondritis results in thickening of the tracheal wall on CT
   e) Pulmonary involvement does not occur in CREST syndrome

28 **In which of the following conditions may diffuse ground glass attenuation be seen on HRCT?**
   a) Pulmonary haemorrhage
   b) Extrinsic allergic alveolitis
   c) Langerhans' cell histiocytosis
   d) Acute respiratory distress syndrome
   e) Asian panbronchiolitis

29 **Which of the following are true regarding chronic eosinophilic pneumonia?**
   a) It has an association with bronchial asthma
   b) It is usually associated with markedly raised immunoglobulin levels
   c) Migratory peripheral consolidations affecting predominantly the lower lobes are typical
   d) Pleural effusions are seen in more than 50% of cases
   e) Unlike acute eosinophilic pneumonia, it is usually not responsive to steroid treatment

30 **Which of the following are true regarding extrinsic allergic alveolitis?**
   a) Ground glass attenuation with areas of lobular sparing is typical on HRCT
   b) The precipitin test is usually negative
   c) Pleural effusions are common
   d) Bronchiectasis occurs in chronic disease
   e) Interstitial fibrosis usually affects the lower lobes

31 **Which of the following are true regarding the appearance of sarcoidosis on HRCT?**
   a) Isolated involvement of posterior mediastinal lymph nodes is common
   b) Nodules have a typical bronchovascular distribution
   c) Subpleural nodules are unusual
   d) Thickening of interlobular septae occurs
   e) Mosaic lung attenuation is a well recognised feature

32 **Which of the following are true regarding pulmonary Langerhans' cell histiocytosis in adults?**
   a) Isolated pulmonary involvement is usual
   b) It is strongly associated with cigarette smoking
   c) Thin-walled cysts and bronchocentric nodules are characteristic HRCT features
   d) It has a predilection for the lower lobes
   e) Mediastinal lymphadenopathy is frequently seen

33 Which of the following are true regarding pulmonary alveolar proteinosis?
   a) It occurs most frequently in children
   b) It has an association with lymphoma
   c) It has a characteristic HRCT appearance
   d) It has an increased incidence of *Nocardia* infection
   e) It has a universally poor prognosis

34 Which of the following are true regarding cryptogenic organising pneumonia (COP)?
   a) The disease is rarely symptomatic
   b) An obstructive pattern of lung function impairment is typical
   c) Pleural effusions are common
   d) Bilateral basal peripheral consolidation is a common radiographic finding
   e) Radiographic clearing occurs following steroid treatment

35 Expiratory HRCT of the thorax may be useful when which of the following conditions are suspected?
   a) COP
   b) Bronchiolitis obliterans
   c) Bronchial asthma
   d) Sarcoidosis
   e) Langerhans' cell histiocytosis

36 The 'halo sign' on HRCT may be observed in which of the following conditions?
   a) Invasive aspergillosis
   b) Metastatic choriocarcinoma
   c) Wegener's granulomatosis
   d) Bronchoalveolar cell carcinoma
   e) Sarcoidosis

37 Which of the following are smoking-related disorders?
   a) Bronchogenic carcinoma
   b) Respiratory bronchiolitis-interstitial lung disease (RB-ILD)
   c) Desquamative interstitial pneumonia (DIP)
   d) Pulmonary histiocytosis
   e) Centrilobular emphysema

38 Which of the following are true regarding bronchial artery embolisation for uncontrolled haemoptysis?
   a) The spinal artery of Adamkiewicz should always be identified before embolisation
   b) Embolisation coils should be deployed at the origin of the hypertrophied bronchial artery
   c) Abdominal pain is a known complication
   d) Control of massive haemoptysis is achieved in only 20% of cases
   e) If a rebleed occurs, a repeat embolisation is unlikely to be successful

39 Which of the following are true regarding blunt pulmonary trauma?
   a) Pulmonary contusions show radiographic resolution in 48 hours
   b) Bronchial rupture is always accompanied by pneumothorax
   c) A normal chest radiograph has a good negative predictive value for aortic rupture
   d) Traumatic diaphragmatic rupture is more common on the left side
   e) Aortic rupture most commonly occurs at the aortic root

40 Which of the following are true regarding pulmonary changes after bone marrow transplantation?
   a) Fungal infection is common in the neutropenic phase following transplantation
   b) Patients are most susceptible to bacterial infection in the post-neutropenic phase of transplantation
   c) Lung involvement is common in an acute graft versus host reaction
   d) Cytomegalovirus is the most common cause of pneumonia
   e) Development of obliterative bronchiolitis following allogenic transplant is associated with a high mortality

Answers

1 a) **False** Air bronchograms may be seen within a tumour, most frequently in bronchoalveolar carcinoma.
  b) **False** A 'popcorn' type of calcification is typical of hamartoma and indicates the nodule is benign. However, amorphous calcification, although unusual, can be seen on CT in up to 7% of lung carcinomas, especially in those greater than 5 cm in size.
  c) **True** Fat is only seen in benign lung lesions such as a hamartoma.
  d) **False** A lobulated outline and corona radiata on CT are typical of carcinoma.
  e) **True** A nodule that is enhanced by less than 15 HU following contrast has a high probability of being benign.

2 a) **False** Patients with stages I–IIIA bronchogenic carcinoma are suitable surgical candidates. Ipsilateral lymphadenopathy represents N1 (hilar) or N2 (mediastinal) nodal disease, which can be present in stage II or III disease.
  b) **True** Malignant pleural effusion indicates T4 disease.
  c) **False** Pericardial resection may be undertaken, although in practical terms the cardiothoracic surgeon may not want to undertake such a risky procedure.
  d) **False** Localised chest wall resection may be undertaken.
  e) **True** Tumour infiltration of the great vessels indicates T4 disease.

3 a) **True** Imaging in the coronal plane allows better assessment of the aorto-pulmonary window.
  b) **False** T1-weighted images allow clear visualisation of the extrapleural fat line. Disruption of the line by the tumour suggests chest wall infiltration.
  c) **True** Superior sulcus tumours are clearly delineated on coronal MRI. MRI can be used to assess invasion of the chest wall, an adjacent rib or the brachial plexus.
  d) **False** MRI is as good as CT in the detection of mediastinal invasion. However, involvement of major mediastinal vessels is better demonstrated on MRI, especially with cardiac gating.
  e) **False** Currently, both CT and MRI use size criteria to predict nodal involvement. However, an MRI lymphography agent (Sinerem), comprised of ultra-small superparamagnetic iron oxide particles, is currently under evaluation. Preliminary results have shown a higher sensitivity in detecting abnormal nodes based on signal characteristics following administration of the contrast.

4 **All true** Malignant causes of SVCO are more common than benign causes. The malignant diseases associated with SVCO are bronchogenic carcinoma (especially small-cell carcinoma) and lymphoma. Benign causes include fibrosing mediastinitis, retrosternal goitre, ascending aortic aneurysm, central venous catheter and constrictive pericarditis.

5 a) **True** There is an increased incidence with systemic sclerosis, parenchymal scarring and interstitial inflammation.

   b) **True** The localised form is more common than the diffuse form. Spontaneous radiographic improvement is known to occur after episodes of bronchorrhoea.

   c) **True** Consolidation, associated with small cystic lucent areas giving a bubbly appearance, is typical on CT. CT may also demonstrate air bronchograms and pleural tags.

   d) **False** Pleural effusions are reportedly seen in 8%–30% of cases.

   e) **True** Bronchoalveolar carcinoma is a known cause of a negative PET scan.

6 a) **False** The chest radiograph is abnormal at presentation in 90% of cases because of the endobronchial growth of the tumour. Carcinoid most frequently arises within the central airways, but carcinoid arising in the lung periphery is more likely to be malignant.

   b) **False** Segmental collapse is the most usual radiographic abnormality, but the central tumour can be seen in up to 25% of cases. It has been described as a 'collar-button' tumour because of its extraluminal extension. Calcifications are seen in 33% of cases.

   c) **True** Bronchial carcinoids may secrete adrenocorticotropic hormone (ACTH) resulting in Cushing's syndrome.

   d) **False** Carcinoid syndrome is rare with bronchial carcinoid tumour and usually occurs with associated liver metastases.

   e) **True** Atypical carcinoid metastasises in 50% of cases, most frequently to the hilar lymph nodes. Haematogenous metastasis occurs less frequently.

7 a) **True** Squamous cell carcinoma presents as a central perihilar mass in 65% of cases.

   b) **True** Squamous cell carcinoma may result in ectopic ADH, ACTH, growth hormone (GH) or parathyroid hormone (PTH) production.

   c) **True** Cavitation may be seen in approximately 20% of cases.

   d) **False** Small-cell lung carcinoma metastasises more frequently than squamous cell carcinoma.

   e) **False** Although any cell type may occur, adenocarcinoma is the most common histological type in Pancoast tumour.

8 a) **False** Benign calcification is seen in 10% of hamartomas, and popcorn calcification is typical.

   b) **False** Pulmonary chondroma, gastric leiomyoma and extra-adrenal paraganglioma constitute Carney's triad. The triad has a female preponderance.

   c) **False** Primary pulmonary lymphoma is frequently non-Hodgkin's type, although Hodgkin's disease is still more common in the thorax.

   d) **True** An attenuation value of 200 HU indicates calcification, and calcific masses in the thorax are frequently benign.

   e) **True** Pulmonary involvement is more common in primary amyloidosis. Tracheobronchial masses are more common than parenchymal involvement. Parenchymal lesions present as multiple nodules, with calcifications in about 20% of cases.

9 a) **False** Lymphadenopathy in thoracic lymphoma is commonly bilateral but asymmetrical.

b) **False** The anterior and middle mediastinal lymph nodes are most frequently involved. Posterior mediastinal lymph nodes are rarely enlarged, but when these are involved there is often contiguous nodal enlargement in the retroperitoneum.

c) **True** Pulmonary involvement is frequently perihilar or juxtamediastinal.

d) **True** Pleural effusion is usually the result of lymphatic obstruction secondary to hilar/mediastinal lymphadenopathy.

e) **True** Even with successful chemotherapy, lymph node masses may not resolve completely. Reduction in the activity of a lymph node group on ^{67}gallium scan indicates a response to treatment.

10 a) **False** Unlike malignant mesothelioma, this is not related to asbestos exposure.

b) **True** Hypertrophic osteoarthropathy occurs in 4%–12% of cases.

c) **False** Symptomatic hypoglycaemia occurs in 6% of patients.

d) **False** Calcification is rare.

e) **True** Pedunculation occurs in 50% of benign pleural fibromas.

11 a) **False** Nodular thickening of both the parietal and visceral pleura is usual, although asbestos plaques are typically found along the parietal pleura.

b) **True** Circumferential thickening of the pleura encasing the lung is common.

c) **True** Hypertrophic osteoarthropathy occurs less commonly compared with benign pleural fibroma.

d) **True** Pleural effusions are common and may be haemorrhagic.

e) **True** Invasion of the chest wall, ribs, pericardium, mediastinum and diaphragm is seen in 11%–18% of cases at presentation. Distant metastases are relatively uncommon.

12 All true Common causes of multiple pleural masses include metastases (frequently adenocarcinoma from lung, breast, stomach and ovary primaries) and pleural spread of malignant thymoma and lymphoma. Other more unusual causes include splenosis, amyloidosis, multiple pleural fibromas and other neoplasms.

13 a) **True** Metastatic transitional cell carcinoma may appear as a thin-wall cyst/pneumatocoele following chemotherapy. This can also be seen with treated testicular germ-cell tumours.

b) **False** Miliary metastases are most commonly seen with thyroid and renal cell carcinoma, but may also occur with melanoma, bone sarcoma and choriocarcinoma.

c) **True** Endobronchial metastases may result from renal cell, breast, thyroid, and rectal carcinoma.

d) **True** Lymphangitis carcinomatosa may result from lung, breast, pancreas, gastric, colonic and prostatic carcinoma.

e) **False** Osteosarcoma is the most common cause of calcifying lung metastases. Metastases from colon, thyroid, breast and ovary may rarely calcify.

14 a) **False** The overall incidence of thymoma in patients with myasthenia gravis is 10%–20%. However, about 40% of patients with thymoma have myasthenia gravis.

b) **True** Hypogammaglobulinaemia is seen in 10% of patients. There is also an association with red cell aplasia (5%).

c) **True** Calcification is seen commonly on both radiographs and CT.

d) **False** Invasive thymoma may spread into the mediastinum or pleural space, but haematogenous metastases are rare.

e) **False** The tumour occurs rarely in patients aged less than 20 years, but is equally common in males and females.

15 a) **False** The disease typically affects young adults and may be of two types: hyaline vascular type, or plasma cell type.

b) **True** Uniform intensely enhancing lymphadenopathy is typical, especially in the more common hyaline vascular form of Castleman's disease.

c) **True** Nodal calcification is common on CT.

d) **False** Nodal cavitation is not a feature.

e) **True** Lymphadenopathy may involve the neck or retroperitoneum.

16 a) **False** Unlike chickenpox pneumonia, miliary tuberculosis does not heal with calcifications.

b) **True** Although uncommon, calcified broncholiths can form within airways, resulting in distal atelectasis.

c) **False** Pleural effusions and lymphadenopathy are more common in primary tuberculosis. Cavitation is the cardinal feature of post-primary tuberculosis.

d) **True** CT with multiplanar re-format and 3D-volume rendering techniques is superior to bronchoscopy, as it allows accurate estimation of the length of the stricture, and also provides assessment of the lung distal to the stricture.

e) **True** Branching y or v densities ('tree-in-bud') are a sign of endobronchial spread of infection and indicate active disease. Endobronchial dissemination of disease is frequently encountered in post-primary tuberculosis.

17 a) **False** Round pneumonia occurs most frequently in children in the first decade of life.

b) **False** It is usually observed in the lower lobes, often abutting the pleural surface. Air-bronchograms may be visible within the mass.

c) **False** *Streptococcus pneumoniae* is the most common pathogen. Other reported associations include *Legionella* infection, Q fever, *Haemophilus influenzae* and fungal infection.

d) **False** Round pneumonia often evolves rapidly over a few days into segmental consolidation. Cavitation is unusual.

e) **True** Round pneumonia is a recognised feature of Q-fever infection.

18 a) **False** Viral pneumonia rarely cavitates. Cavitating pneumonia most frequently results from staphylococcal, streptococcal and *Klebsiella* infections.

b) **True** Pulmonary gangrene is a rare complication of *Klebsiella* pneumonia, secondary to severe necrosis.

c) **False** *Chlamydia* pneumonia is frequently nonsegmental and is rarely associated with effusions.

d) **False** Perihilar consolidation associated with hilar lymphadenopathy is frequently seen in pertussis pneumonia.

e) **True** Obliterative bronchiolitis, resulting in air trapping and mosaic attenuation on CT, is a known complication of *Mycoplasma* infection.

19 a) **True**

b) **True**

c) **False**

d) **False**

e) **True**

Calcification of lymph nodes is a feature of sarcoidosis and silicosis and is seen on radiographs in 5% of patients. The incidence of calcification is higher on CT. Other causes of nodal calcifications include coal miner's pneumoconiosis, lymphoma following treatment, amyloidosis and *P. carinii* infection. Asbestosis and berylliosis do not result in nodal calcification.

20 a) **False** Acute silicoproteinosis occurs from intense exposure to silica dust, resulting in an alveolar exudate, which has mid-zone and upper-zone predominance.

b) **True** On HRCT, silicosis appears as multiple small, 2–5 mm centrilobular or subpleural nodules, often with posterior-zone and upper-zone predominance. Nodal enlargement may be present. The appearance on HRCT can mimic sarcoidosis.

c) **True** Progressive massive fibrosis develops on a background of diffuse lung nodules and usually has an irregular border with adjacent parenchymal distortion and cicatricial emphysema.

d) **True** Nodal calcification is seen on the radiograph in 5% of patients with silicosis compared with 1% of patients with coal miner's pneumoconiosis.

(e) **False** Impairment of the lung function test correlates best with the degree of emphysematous change. Nodular profusion is a weaker independent correlate.

21 a) **True** Asbestos-related pleural plaques occur along the parietal pleura, with a predilection for the diaphragmatic surface and along the posterolateral chest wall in the mid-zone and lower zones. Sparing of the costophrenic recess and mediastinal surface is characteristic.

b) **False** Pleural plaques may extend into interlobular fissures.

c) **True** Benign isolated pleural effusion is common in the asbestos-exposed population and is a diagnosis made by exclusion.

d) **True** On HRCT, subpleural fibrosis is typical, with thickened interlobular septae, honeycomb change, pleural thickening, subpleural line and parenchymal bands.

e) **False** Asbestosis is associated with pleural plaques in 80% of cases.

22 a) False Rounded atelectasis appears as a well defined oval or rounded mass, which has a subpleural location, usually in the posterior or basal region of the lower lobes.

b) True An acute angle with the pleural margin is typical, indicating its intrapulmonary location.

c) True Pleural thickening near the rounded atelectasis is typical.

d) True Crowding of the vasculature results in the comet tail appearance, which refers to the curvilinear bronchi and vessels seen entering the mass. Usually there is also volume loss within the affected lobe, with inferior migration of the interlobar fissure.

e) False On CT, the mass enhances uniformly with intravenous contrast.

23 a) True The severity of lung changes following radiotherapy is related to the volume of lung irradiated, the total and fractionated radiation dose, previous or concomitant treatment (e.g. chemotherapy) and individual susceptibility.

b) False Acute radiation pneumonitis is characteristically restricted to the involved field. The earliest change appears at 6–8 weeks after the beginning of treatment, reaching a peak at 3–4 months.

c) False Pleural effusion is rare, occurring in the acute phase.

d) False Radiation fibrosis develops over 12–18 months following radiotherapy; often associated with parenchymal distortion and traction bronchiectasis.

e) True Pulmonary oligaemia is a late feature resulting from vascular sclerosis leading to diminished perfusion.

24 a) False UIP has no gender predilection.

b) True The majority of the cases of cryptogenic fibrosing alveolitis result from UIP.

c) True The peak incidence is in the fifth and sixth decades of life.

d) True Areas of ground glass attenuation on HRCT without parenchymal distortion indicate active alveolitis, which may be reversible with steroid treatment. Ground glass attenuation associated with parenchymal distortion usually signifies established fibrosis.

e) False The characteristic temporal heterogeneity on HRCT allows a confident diagnosis to be made in the large proportion of cases. Temporal heterogeneity refers to different areas of lung, demonstrating different stages of inflammation and fibrosis at the same time.

25 a) True Pleural effusion usually occurs in long-standing disease, with a male preponderance (M:F = 9:1). Effusions are bilateral in 20% of cases and are commonly associated with the presence of cutaneous nodules.

b) False Rheumatoid lung nodules are usually associated with established arthritis, although they may occur with or before the onset of arthritis. They are also more common in men and up to 80% are associated with cutaneous nodules.

c) False Rheumatoid nodules may be single (25%) or multiple (75%), usually in the upper zones or mid zones of the lungs, and 50% cavitate.

d) True Other findings of increased frequency in rheumatoid lungs include bronchiectasis, cryptogenic organising pneumonia (COP), pulmonary fibrosis, obliterative bronchiolitis and follicular bronchiolitis.

e) True Mosaic lung attenuation results from small airway disease (obliterative bronchiolitis). This may be related to the disease itself or be a consequence of treatment with gold/penicillamine.

26 a) **True**   Primary pleural effusion in SLE is frequently painful and associated with pleuritis. Effusions commonly occur in 20%–30% of patients.

   b) **True**   SLE is associated with the presence of lupus anticoagulant, which increases the incidence of thromboembolic disease.

   c) **True**   Diaphragmatic dysfunction manifests as a raised hemidiaphragm on the chest radiograph.

   d) **False**   Death usually results from renal failure or cerebral lupus.

   e) **False**   Infection is the most common cause of air space shadowing within the lungs. Pulmonary haemorrhage is associated with active disease and is associated with a very high mortality rate (70%).

27 a) **True**   Aspiration pneumonia is the most common radiographic abnormality in patients with polymyositis or dermatomyositis. This results from pharyngeal weakness and defective swallowing mechanism. Other lung changes include interstitial fibrosis, pulmonary arterial hypertension and diaphragmatic weakness.

   b) **False**   Pleural effusions and pleuritis are common. However, fine interstitial fibrosis is frequently seen on HRCT.

   c) **True**   There is a higher incidence of lymphocytic interstitial pneumonia and lymphoma in patients with Sjögren's syndrome.

   d) **True**   On CT, relapsing polychondritis results in thickening, expansion and calcification of the tracheal cartilage, with narrowing of the lumen. This later results in stricture formation.

   e) **False**   Pulmonary fibrosis occurs but the incidence is lower in CREST syndrome compared with systemic sclerosis.

28 a) **True**

   b) **True**

   c) **False**

   d) **True**

   e) **False**

       Ground glass opacification refers to increased attenuation of the lung on HRCT, without obscuring the visibility of the pulmonary vasculature and bronchioles. This appearance can result from the presence of fluid, blood, pus, or cells within the acini. The causes include pulmonary oedema, fluid overload, pulmonary haemorrhage, acute respiratory distress syndrome, sarcoidosis, extrinsic allergic alveolitis, alveolar proteinosis and alveolar cell carcinoma. Langerhans' cell histiocytosis is characterised by cysts and nodules. Asian panbronchiolitis results in a proliferative bronchiolitis, giving rise to widespread 'tree-in-bud' opacities.

29 a) **True**   40% of patients have a history of asthma and 50% are atopic.

   b) **False**   The serum IgE levels are usually normal, allowing differentiation from conditions associated with raised serum IgE levels, such as allergic bronchopulmonary aspergillosis and parasite-associated eosinophilic lung syndromes.

   c) **False**   Peripheral, nonsegmental consolidation in the upper or mid zones is typical, occurring in two-thirds of cases.

   d) **False**   Pleural effusion is uncommon (2%).

   e) **False**   The condition is steroid responsive, clearing rapidly over days. However, relapse is common.

30 a) **True** Ground glass attenuation with lobular sparing is typical, giving rise to a mosaic pattern on HRCT. Bronchiolitis is also associated, resulting in lobular air trapping, which contributes to the mosaic attenuation pattern.

b) **False** The precipitin test is frequently positive. However, a positive precipitin merely indicates exposure to the antigen, and not necessarily the cause of the disease.

c) **False** Pleural changes are not a feature of the disease.

d) **True** Parenchymal distortion and traction bronchiectasis result from interstitial fibrosis, which occurs in chronic disease.

e) **False** Fibrotic changes usually involve the upper lobes.

31 a) **False** Posterior mediastinal lymph nodes are least frequently involved in sarcoidosis. Hilar, right paratracheal and subcarinal lymph nodes are most frequently involved. Anterior mediastinal lymph nodes may be enlarged, but not usually in isolation.

b) **True** Pulmonary nodules have a bronchovascular distribution, resulting in beading of the bronchovascular interstitium on HRCT.

c) **False** Nodules have a predilection for the subpleural location, appearing as beading of the pleura and interlobular septae.

d) **True** Sarcoidosis is a cause of thickening of the interlobular septae.

e) **True** Mosaic lung attenuation reflecting small airway involvement is one of the earliest signs of lung involvement by sarcoidosis and can precede the appearance of intrapulmonary nodules.

32 a) **True** Unlike childhood Langerhans' cell histiocytosis, adult pulmonary Langerhans' cell histiocytosis is usually confined to the chest.

b) **True** There is a definite association with smoking. Cessation of smoking frequently leads to radiological improvement of the disease.

c) **True** Thin-walled irregular cysts and bronchocentric nodules are typical features on HRCT. Frequently, the costophrenic angle and lung apices are spared.

d) **False** It has a predilection for the upper zones of the lungs.

e) **False** Mediastinal lymphadenopathy is infrequently encountered.

33 a) **False** Although the peak incidence occurs in the fourth and fifth decades, the condition can occur at any age. There is an increased incidence in males.

b) **True** The condition is frequently idiopathic, but may be associated with lymphoma, haematological disorders and immune suppression.

c) **True** The characteristic HRCT appearance is geographical ground glass opacification, associated with thickening of the interlobular septae, giving rise to a crazypaving appearance.

d) **True** It is associated with an increased incidence of *Nocardia* infection.

e) **False** About 50% of patients show improvement or remission with bronchoalveolar lavage.

34 a) **False** COP is also known as bronchiolitis obliterans organising pneumonia (BOOP) or bronchiolitis obliterans with intramural polyps. The peak incidence is in the fifth and sixth decades of life, with equal gender predisposition. About 50% of patients are symptomatic, presenting with fever, cough, breathlessness and malaise.

b) **True** The presence of intramural polyps results in a predominantly obstructive pattern on lung function tests.

c) **False** Pleural effusions are uncommon, occurring in less than 5% of cases.

d) **True** The typical radiographic appearance is one of multiple, bilateral, asymmetric consolidation, with a basal and peripheral predominance, accompanied by nodules and reticular change.

e) **True** The condition is usually steroid responsive, resolving in days to weeks following treatment. However, relapse is not infrequent following steroid withdrawal.

35 a) **False** COP is characterised by peripheral basal consolidation. Air trapping is not a dominant feature.

b) **True** Expiratory scans are helpful in conditions resulting in constrictive bronchiolitis and air trapping. The visualisation of air trapping in the pulmonary lobules is enhanced on expiratory scans.

c) **True** Minor thickening of the airways may occur in bronchial asthma. However, the degree of air trapping is best appreciated on expiratory scans.

d) **True** Small airway involvement occurs early in pulmonary sarcoidosis, resulting in air trapping and mosaic lung attenuation.

e) **False** Langerhans' cell histiocytosis does not result in airway abnormality. Hence, expiratory scans are unhelpful.

36 a) **True**

b) **True**

c) **True**

d) **True**

e) **False**

The 'halo' sign refers to the increase in lung attenuation surrounding a lung lesion. The appearance can be seen in invasive aspergillosis, which is a result of hyphae infiltration into the lung parenchyma. The phenomenon is a result of perilesional haemorrhage in metastatic choriocarcinoma and Wegener's granulomatosis. Alveolar spread of bronchoalveolar cell carcinoma results in the appearance of a 'halo' in these patients.

37 All true All these conditions are related to smoking. RB-ILD and DIP occur as a response to cigarette smoke, resulting in accumulation of 'pigmented' macrophages within the respiratory bronchioles and the adjacent alvioli. In RB-ILD, the lung involvement is typically centred on the small airways, and is characterised on HRCT by a background of ground-glass attenuation with superimposed centrilobular nodules. Septal lines and emphysematous change may be present. The lung changes are similar in DIP, except that the disease tends to affect the lung more uniformally and diffusely. On HRCT, diffuse ground-glass attenuation is frequently seen in the mid and lower zones and may show a subplural prediction. It may be difficult to distinguishable RB-ILD from DIP on imaging and histopathology.

38 a) **False** Failure to visualise the spinal artery should not be a contraindication to embolisation. Preferential flow into the hypertrophied bronchial vessels frequently occurs and the spinal artery may not be easily visualised. However, if the spinal artery is seen arising from a bronchial artery, then caution should be taken when performing the embolisation.

b) **False** Embolisation may be performed using particles, gel-foam and coils. A metallic coil should not be deployed at the origin of the bronchial artery, as it would preclude further embolisation if necessary.

c) **True** Spillover of embolic material into the thoracic aorta can result in intestinal ischaemia, causing abdominal pain.

d) **False** Initial control of haemoptysis is achieved in 70%–80% of cases. However, there is a rebleed rate of 20% in the following 6 months.

e) **False** Rebleed in patients can be successfully treated with embolisation.

39 a) **True** Pulmonary contusions, which appear as airspace opacification over the site of trauma, resolve rapidly, usually within 48 hours.

b) **False** Bronchial rupture is frequently (70%), but not invariably, associated with a pneumothorax. The falling lung sign, referring to the displacement of the lung to the dependent position, is typical.

c) **True** A normal chest radiograph has a 98% negative predictive value for significant intrathoracic injury.

d) **True** Traumatic diaphragmatic injury is more common on the left side. MRI has the highest sensitivity in the detection of diaphragmatic injury.

e) **False** Aortic rupture is most common at the level of the ductus arteriosus.

40 a) **True** The pre-engraftment (neutropenic) phase following bone marrow transplant (up to 30 days) is characterised by severe neutropenia. At this time, patients are most susceptible to bacteria and fungal infections.

b) **False** The post-engraftment (post-neutropenic) phase occurs at about 30–100 days following transplantation. At this stage, neutropenia is recovering, but there is still considerable depressed lymphocytic humoral and cellular immunity. Viral and protozoal infections are most common at this stage.

c) **False** Acute graft versus host reactions occur with allogenic transplants, usually affecting the gastrointestinal tract, liver and skin. Involvement of the lungs is rare. A chronic graft versus host reaction is a more systemic disease with lung involvement.

d) **True** Overall, infection due to cytomegalovirus accounts for up to 50% of infections encountered in bone marrow transplant patients.

e) **True** Obliterative bronchiolitis occurs in the late stages of post-allogeneic bone marrow transplantation and has a 50% mortality rate. The condition responds poorly to steroids.

Chapter 2

Cardiovascular imaging

1   **Which of the following statements are true?**
    a)   In interruption of the inferior vena cava (IVC), the hepatic veins drain directly
         into the right atrium
    b)   The pulmonary arteries cannot be differentiated from adjacent bronchi
         with gradient echo magnetic resonance imaging (MRI)
    c)   A left-sided superior vena cava (SVC) occurs in 10% of the population
    d)   The anomalous right-sided subclavian artery indents the anterior surface
         of the oesophagus
    e)   A ratio of ascending to descending aortic diameter at the level of the aortic
         root of greater than 1.7 is abnormal

2   **Regarding aortic transection (traumatic aortic injury), which of the following are true?**
    a)   The most common site is the ascending aorta
    b)   The descending aorta is rarely involved
    c)   The 'left apical cap' sign is highly specific for aortic transection
    d)   The chest radiograph is normal in 30% of cases at presentation
    e)   Chronic false aneurysm develops in 5% of cases

3   **In cardiac MRI, which of the following are true?**
    a)   The normal pericardium returns low signal on T1-weighted imaging
    b)   Prosthetic heart valves are an absolute contraindication to MRI scanning
    c)   The superior pericardial recess is rarely seen on MRI
    d)   In constrictive pericarditis, the pericardium is typically thickened
    e)   MRI may distinguish constrictive pericarditis from restrictive cardiomyopathy

4   **Which of the following are true regarding pericardial defects?**
    a)   The left side is most commonly affected
    b)   They are associated with bronchogenic cysts
    c)   Most patients are symptomatic
    d)   Tracheal deviation is a typical feature on chest radiography
    e)   Surgical treatment is indicated in the majority

5   **Regarding Takayasu's arteritis, which of the following are true?**
    a)   Males are more commonly affected than females
    b)   The erythrocyte sedimentation rate (ESR) is rarely elevated
    c)   The left subclavian artery is rarely involved
    d)   Pulmonary arteries are commonly involved
    e)   Aortic calcification is a feature on chest radiography in 40% of cases

6   **Which of the following are true regarding transposition of the great arteries (TGA)?**
    a)   In the D loop of TGA, the atria and ventricles have a normal morphological relationship
    b)   Pulmonary stenosis is an associated feature
    c)   Chest radiograph shows pulmonary plethora in the D loop of TGA
    d)   In the L loop (corrected) transposition, there is a physiologically corrected circulation
    e)   Dextrocardia is associated with the L loop of TGA

7   **In tetralogy of Fallot, which of the following are true?**
a)   Pulmonary artery hypoplasia is an associated finding
b)   Right-sided aortic arch is present in 5% of cases
c)   Right ventricular hypertrophy is a feature of antenatal scanning at midtrimester
d)   The most common associated coronary artery variant is an anomalous origin of the left anterior descending artery
e)   The aortic root over-rides the ventriculoseptal defect

8   **Regarding total anomalous pulmonary venous drainage (TAPVD), which of the following are true?**
a)   The supracardiac type is the most common
b)   The left atrium is not enlarged
c)   The infracardiac type may drain into the hepatic veins
d)   Pulmonary oedema in the presence of a normal size heart is a feature of cardiac type TAPVD
e)   There is an association with scimitar syndrome

9   **Which of the following are true regarding aortic dissection?**
a)   There is an association with Turner's syndrome
b)   Cardiac failure is a common presenting feature
c)   The most common site in the ascending aorta is the left lateral wall
d)   Chest radiograph shows a left pleural effusion in 30% of cases
e)   The aortic intimal flap is seen in 75% of cases at angiography

10   **Regarding the pulmonary arteries, which of the following are true?**
a)   The upper lobe pulmonary veins lie lateral to the upper lobe arteries on chest radiography
b)   On a lateral chest radiograph, the right pulmonary artery lies posterosuperior to the carina
c)   The pulmonary artery systolic pressure may be estimated by Doppler echocardiography
d)   Pulmonary arteriovenous malformations are rarely multiple
e)   A pulmonary varix is commonly found in the upper lobes

11   **Which of the following are true regarding inflammatory aneurysm of the abdominal aorta?**
a)   Periaortic fibrosis usually appears as a well defined soft tissue mass
b)   Fibrosis typically spares the posterior aorta
c)   Extension into the pelvis is a feature
d)   On computed tomography (CT), periaortic fibrosis enhances avidly following intravenous contrast
e)   On MRI, periaortic fibrosis gives typically high signal on T1-weighted imaging

12   **In patients following thoracotomy, which of the following are true?**
a)   Mediastinal infection has a mortality rate of 25%
b)   Postoperative haematoma usually resolves on CT after 2–3 weeks
c)   Pericardial effusion is not a normal finding following sternotomy
d)   Mediastinal air usually resolves within 7 days
e)   CT is the technique of choice in establishing the diagnosis of mediastinitis

13 Which of the following are true regarding the cardiopulmonary system during pregnancy?
a) Cardiac output may increase by 85% during delivery
b) In peripartum cardiomyopathy, cardiac size can predict prognosis
c) Amniotic fluid embolism may be associated with disseminated intravascular coagulation (DIC)
d) Spontaneous pneumothorax during pregnancy is common
e) Cardiac activity is visualised by transvaginal scan when crown-to-rump length (CRL) is 5 mm

14 Which of the following are true regarding MRI and heart disease?
a) Infarcted myocardium is typically high signal on T2-weighted imaging
b) There is marked enhancement of infarcted myocardium following intravenous gadolinium contrast
c) The cardiac valves are well demonstrated on MRI
d) In acute myocardial infarction, systolic wall thickening is reduced
e) Viable myocardium may be differentiated from infarcted tissue

15 Regarding cardiac myxomas, which of the following are true?
a) 20% of patients are asymptomatic
b) Embolism occurs in 20% of patients
c) The most common site is the right atrium
d) It is usually homogenous in attenuation on contrast-enhanced CT
e) There is an association with myxoid fibroadenomas of the breast

16 Which of the following are true regarding benign cardiac tumours?
a) Papillary fibroelastomas typically affect the ventricles
b) Recurrence after excision of papillary fibroelastomas is common
c) Rhabdomyomas of the heart are typically seen in children aged less than 1 year
d) Rhabdomyoma is associated with tuberous sclerosis
e) Cardiomegaly is the most common radiological finding in patients with cardiac fibroma(s)

17 Regarding aortic aneurysms, which of the following are true?
a) Abdominal aortic aneurysm is associated with renal artery stenosis (RAS) in 25% of cases
b) Abdominal aortic aneurysm extends to involve the common iliac arteries in 65% of cases
c) Mycotic aneurysm most frequently affects the ascending aorta
d) Thoracic aortic aneurysm is the most common vascular cause of a mediastinal mass
e) Renal failure occurs in 14% of postoperative patients

18 In Buerger's disease, which of the following are true?
a) There is a strong association with cigarette smoking
b) Raynaud's phenomenon occurs in 30% of cases
c) The upper limbs are more frequently affected than the lower limbs
d) Migratory thrombophlebitis is an associated feature
e) There is typically tapered narrowing of the occluded artery

19 Which of the following are true regarding coarctation of the aorta?
a) Adult coarctation is commonly associated with cardiac anomalies
b) The ductus arteriosus usually remains patent in adult type coarctation
c) A short segment of narrowing of the ascending aorta is seen in infantile coarctation
d) It is a rare cause of infantile heart failure
e) Rib notching is usually present by 1 year of age

20 Which of the following are true regarding splenic abnormalities?
a) Polysplenia is associated with left-sided azygos continuation of an interrupted IVC
b) Gastrointestinal malrotation is associated with polysplenia
c) Asplenia is rarely associated with total anomalous pulmonary venous drainage
d) Duplex kidneys are seen in the majority of patients with asplenia
e) Howell–Jolly bodies in the peripheral blood are a feature of asplenia

Answers

1 a) **True**   The IVC terminates before reaching the right atrium and blood reaches the SVC via the azygos vein on the right side. The hepatic veins drain directly into the right atrium. This is a rare anomaly and usually does not produce symptoms. It is associated with polysplenia syndrome, asplenia syndrome, dextrocardia and a retroaortic left renal vein.

   b) **False**   Blood returns high signal from within the arteries on gradient echo sequences, allowing differentiation from adjacent bronchi, unless saturation bands have been applied.

   c) **False**   Left-sided SVC is seen in 0.3% of the population and 4% of patients with congenital heart disease.

   d) **False**   The anomalous right-sided subclavian artery arises from the descending portion of the aortic arch and is the last of the great vessels to arise from this point. It passes to the right, posterior to the oesophagus.

   e) **True**   A ratio greater than 1.7 indicates aortic root dilatation.

2 a) **False**   The most common site is the aortic isthmus (95% of cases). The ascending aorta is involved in only 1% of cases.

   b) **True**   The descending aorta is rarely involved (2% of cases).

   c) **False**   The 'left apical cap' is a sign of mediastinal haematoma with extrapleural extension of blood (but only 15% of cases of mediastinal haematoma are due to an aortic tear).

   d) **True**   A delay of up to 36 hours may occur before the onset of radiographic signs.

   e) **True**   Chronic aortic pseudoaneurysm occurs in 5% of patients who survive aortic transection. Patients may be symptom free for years and present with delayed symptoms. Complications include progressive dilatation and rupture, bacterial endocarditis, lumen obstruction and aorto-oesophageal fistula.

3 a) **True**   The pericardium consists of predominantly fibrous tissue, which returns low signal.

   b) **False**   Most cardiac valves (except the old Star Edwards) are MRI compatible.

   c) **False**   The superior pericardial recess is usually seen on MRI.

   d) **True**   In constrictive pericarditis, MRI shows a thickened pericardium (greater than 5 mm) with a small right ventricle with decreased end-diastolic volume.

   e) **True**   See d) above. In restrictive cardiomyopathy, the pericardium is typically normal and an associated small pericardial effusion and abnormal myocardial systolic thickening may be seen.

4 a) **True** Part of the pericardium develops poorly due to premature atrophy of the cardinal vein, which leads to loss of integrity of the pleuropericardial membrane. The left side is affected in 70% of cases and total bilateral absence is seen in 9%.

b) **True** Other associations include ventriculoseptal defect, patent ductus arteriosus, diaphragmatic hernia and mitral stenosis.

c) **False** Symptoms when present may include palpitations, tachycardia, syncope and chest pain. However, most patients are asymptomatic.

d) **False** Tracheal deviation is not a feature. Radiographic findings are only present with large defects or complete pericardial absence and include poor definition of the right heart border with levoposition and absence of the left pericardial fat pad.

e) **False** Surgical treatment is not indicated in the majority, but may, however, be required when there is herniation of the atria or the atrial appendage.

5 a) **False** Females are more commonly affected than males (M:F = 1:8).

b) **False** ESR is typically elevated in 80% of cases.

c) **False** Takayasu's arteritis is a chronic arteritis, which affects the aortic segments and their branches. The left subclavian, common carotid and brachiocephalic trunk, coeliac axis, superior mesenteric artery and pulmonary arteries are commonly affected. The axillary, vertebral and brachial arteries are rarely involved.

d) **True** See c) above.

e) **False** Aortic calcification is seen in 15% of cases. Other chest radiography features include widened mediastinum, focal pulmonary oligaemia and abnormal descending aortic contour.

6 a) **True** In the D loop of TGA, the aorta arises from the right ventricle and the pulmonary artery from the left ventricle. A normal relationship exists between the atria and the ventricles. TGA have a normal anterior–posterior relationship.

b) **True** Other associations include ventriculoseptal defect, patent ductus arteriosus and coarctation of the aorta.

c) **True** Chest radiograph shows cardiomegaly and a narrow pedicle ('egg on a string' appearance), as the aorta lies anterior to the main pulmonary artery.

d) **True** In the L loop of TGA, there is transposition of the aorta and pulmonary arteries in addition to inversion of the left and right ventricles. The atria and coronary arteries are associated with their corresponding ventricles.

e) **True** Dextrocardia with situs solitus (normal situs) is associated with congenital heart disease in 95% of cases. Dextrocardia associated with situs inversus is associated with congenital heart disease in 5% of cases (e.g. Kartagener's syndrome).

7 a) **True** See e) below.

b) **False** Right-sided aortic arch is present in 25% of cases and is usually of the mirror-image type.

c) **False** Antenatal ultrasound findings include dilated over-riding aorta, perimembranous ventricular septal defect and mildly stenotic right ventricular outflow tract, but right ventricular hypertrophy is not a feature at this stage.

d) **True** The left anterior descending artery arises from the right coronary artery and runs over the surface of the ventricle where it may be at risk during surgery.

e) **True** Other features of the tetralogy of Fallot include large ventriculoseptal defect, right ventricular outflow tract stenosis and right ventricular hypertrophy.

8 a) **True** In TAPVD, the pulmonary confluence fails to communicate with the left atrium. In the supracardiac type (52% of cases), the pulmonary confluence drains into an ascending vein on the left (remnant of the leftsided SVC), which in turn drains into the left brachiocephalic vein and subsequently the right sided SVC. In the cardiac type (30% of cases), the abnormality drains via the coronary sinus into the right atrium. In the infracardiac type (12% of cases), the pulmonary confluence drains into a descending vein, which passes through the diaphragm, where it may be obstructed, and into the portal vein, the IVC or the hepatic veins.

b) **True** The right atrium and ventricle have volume overload. An atrial septal defect is critical for survival as it allows the return of oxygenated blood to the systemic circulation. Other radiographic features of the supracardiac type include increased pulmonary blood flow and the characteristic figure-of-eight cardiac silhouette.

c) **True** See a) above.

d) **False** Pulmonary oedema is a characteristic feature of the infracardiac type TAPVD.

e) **False** Scimitar syndrome is the association of hypogenetic lung with congenital pulmonary venolobar syndrome where all or part of the hypogenetic lung is drained via an anomalous vein into the subdiaphragmatic IVC, hepatic veins, portal vein or coronary sinus.

9 a) **True** Other associations include: hypertension in 60%–90% of cases, Marfan's syndrome, relapsing polychondritis, Ehlers–Danlos syndrome and coarctation of the aorta.

b) **False** Cardiac failure is rare at presentation. Common signs include asymmetrical or absent femoral and peripheral pulses, neurological deficits, haemodynamic shock and aortic regurgitation.

c) **False** In the ascending aorta, the most common site of aortic dissection is the anterior and right lateral wall, the superior and posterior wall at the aortic arch and the posterior and left lateral wall of the descending aorta. The ascending aorta and/or the aortic arch are involved in 70% of cases and 30% involve the descending aorta only.

d) **True** Other radiographic features include: inward displacement of atherosclerotic plaque, a difference in size between the ascending and descending aorta, mediastinal widening, cardiac enlargement and left lower lobe atelectasis.

e) **True** Other features at angiography include opacification of two aortic lumens, abnormal placement of catheters, compression of the true lumen by the false lumen and aortic regurgitation.

10 a) **True** The lower lobe veins have a more horizontal course as they lie towards the left atrium.

b) **False** The left pulmonary artery lies posterosuperior to the carina. The right pulmonary artery lies in front and below the carina.

c) **True** Estimation of the pulmonary artery systolic pressure may be achieved by measuring the velocity of the regurgitated jet through the tricuspid valve with Doppler echocardiography.

d) **False** Pulmonary arteriovenous malformations are multiple in one-third of cases and frequently associated with Rendu–Osler–Weber syndrome (60% of cases). However, only 5%–15% of patients with Rendu–Osler–Weber syndrome have pulmonary arteriovenous malformations.

e) **False** A pulmonary varix is a tortuous dilatation of a pulmonary vein just before draining into the left atrium – usually seen in the infrahilar region.

11 a) **True**   This is a variant of the abdominal aortic aneurysm (AAA) when there is inflammatory change in the periaortic tissue. The inflammatory changes are usually well defined and begin anterolaterally, sparing the posterior aortic wall. Occasionally they may be poorly defined and extend along the posterior aortic wall.

    b) **True**   See a) above.

    c) **True**   Extension along the iliac vessels may occur.

    d) **False**   Enhancement after contrast is usually variable, depending on the degree of fibrosis, hyalinisation and lipogranulomatosis.

    e) **False**   The fibrosis usually has low or intermediate signal. The signal on T2-weighted imaging is variable.

12 a) **True**   Diffuse mediastinitis has a mortality rate approaching 50%, but which decreases with early diagnosis.

    b) **True**   Normal findings include: retrosternal soft tissue infiltration with blood or oedema, air, haematoma, bone defects and minimal pericardial thickening.

    c) **False**   Minimal effusion can be normal.

    d) **True**   However, postoperative changes may persist longer than 7 days.

    e) **False**   Although CT plays an essential role, diagnosis is established by microbiological examination. CT may show the extent of the fluid collection and can be used to guide aspiration or drainage.

13 a) **True**   Cardiac output increases more in vaginal than caesarean deliveries. This can result in pulmonary vascular engorgement and left ventricular enlargement.

    b) **True**   Peripartum cardiomyopathy occurs from the last month of pregnancy to 6 months post-partum. Chest radiography findings include cardiac enlargement and pulmonary oedema. Although 80% of cases initially improve, the overall mortality reaches 60%. The heart size at 6 months can predict prognosis.

    c) **True**   Amniotic fluid embolism can occur at delivery or peripartum, especially during prolonged labour. Circulatory shock with extensive haemorrhage occurs due to DIC.

    d) **False**   Spontaneous pneumothorax during pregnancy is rare, but affected individuals tend to have prolonged labour, asthma or a history of pneumothorax.

    e) **True**   Cardiac activity is visualised by transabdominal ultrasonography when CRL is greater than 9 mm (6.9 weeks) and by transvaginal scan when CRL exceeds 5 mm (6.2 weeks).

14 a) **True**   The infarcted area is low signal on T1-weighted imaging.

    b) **True**   Infarcted myocardium may be better visualised on postintravenous gadolinium T1-weighted images compared with T2-weighted images.

    c) **False**   The myocardium and endocardial surface are well demonstrated on MRI. The interatrial and interventricular septae, papillary apparatus and moderator band are generally well seen. The cardiac valves are, however, inconsistently seen.

    d) **True**   Using criteria of systolic wall thickness and abnormally high signal on T2-weighted images, the accuracy of MRI in cardiac infarction is more than 85%.

    e) **True**   Viable myocardium, unlike infarcted tissue, shows wall thickening at systole and thinning at diastole.

15 a) **True** Left atrial myxomas may cause mitral valve obstruction, leading to dyspnoea and orthopnoea due to pulmonary oedema. Right atrial myxoma may obstruct the tricuspid valve and cause right-sided heart failure. The classic triad consists of obstructive cardiac symptoms, embolic phenomena and constitutional symptoms.

   b) **True** Embolism is the second most common feature of cardiac myxomas, frequently involving the central nervous system, coronary arteries, kidney, spleen and pulmonary arteries. It is seen in up to 40% of cases.

   c) **False** The most common site of cardiac myxomas is the left atrium (75% of cases). The ventricles are rarely affected and 20% of tumours occur in the right atrium.

   d) **False** The tumour is low attenuation compared with intracardiac blood and is heterogeneous due to frequent necrosis, haemorrhage, cystic change, fibrosis or ossification.

   e) **True** Most (93%) myxoid fibroadenomas of the breast are sporadic. The remainder may be associated with the autosomal dominant Carney syndrome (skin and myxoid fibroadenomas of the breast, skin pigmentation, pituitary adenomas and testicular tumour).

16 a) **False** Papillary fibroelastomas (benign endocardial papillomas) mainly affect the valves. They are the second most common primary benign cardiac tumour. Most are small when discovered at echocardiography and are not usually associated with valvular malfunction.

   b) **False** Recurrence after excision of papillary fibroelastomas is rare.

   c) **True** Most (90%) rhabdomyomas of the heart occur in children aged less than 1 year. They are benign hamartomas and may be associated with tuberous sclerosis in 50% of cases. At echocardiography, they appear as hyperechoic nodules. When multiple, they may cause diffuse myocardial thickening.

   d) **True** See c) above.

   e) **True** Cardiac fibromas are congenital tumours with 33% occurring in those aged less than 1 year and 15% in adolescents. They may be associated with Gorlin's syndrome. Cardiomegaly and a focal bulge in the cardiac contour are common radiological findings. Calcification is seen in 25% of cases. MRI reveals these tumours to be hyperintense to myocardium and hypointense on T2-weighted images, which is typical of fibrous tissue.

17 a) **True** Stenosis of the coeliac and superior mesenteric artery (SMA) is seen in 22% of cases of abdominal aortic aneurysms and occlusion of the inferior mesenteric artery occurs in 80%.

   b) **True** Most (90%) abdominal aortic aneurysms are infrarenal.

   c) **True** Mycotic aneurysm arises from a variety of non-syphilitic infections (*Staphylococcus aureus*, *Salmonella*, *Neisseria gonorrhoeae*). The ascending aorta is most commonly affected with involvement of the visceral arteries in the abdomen. Most are true aneurysms involving dilatation of all three layers of the aortic wall.

   d) **True** Other vascular causes of a mediastinal mass include: right sided/double aortic arch, anomalous origin of the right subclavian artery, ectatic or dilated subclavian vein, thoracic aorta, aneurysm of the sinus of Valsalva, oesophageal varices and interruption of the IVC with azygos or hemi-azygos continuation.

   e) **True**

18 a) **True**   Buerger's disease is a segmental obliterative vasculitis affecting the medium and small arteries. Veins are affected in 30% of cases. Of those affected, 95% are smokers and 98% are male.

     b) **True**   Other causes of Raynaud's phenomenon include vasculitis, atherosclerosis, drugs (eg, ergot), dysproteinaemia, myxoedema and primary pulmonary hypertension

     c) **False**   Lower limbs are affected (80% of cases) more often than upper limbs

     d) **True**   Migratory thrombophlebitis is seen in up to one third of patients.

     e) **True**   Skip lesions are typical as well as abundant corkscrew collaterals, one of which may follow the path of the original artery (Martorell's sign).

19 a) **False**   Adult coarctation is a short narrowing at the ligamentum arteriosum. It is rarely associated with cardiac anomalies and the ductus arteriosum is usually closed. Angiography shows a shelf-like lesion with prestenotic narrowing and poststenotic dilatation.

     b) **False**   See a) above.

     c) **False**   Infantile aortic coarctation involves a long tubular segment of the aortic arch distal to the origin of the brachiocephalic artery.

     d) **False**   Aortic coarctation is the second most common cause of heart failure in the neonate (hypoplastic left heart is the most common).

     e) **False**   Rib notching involves the third to eighth ribs and in 75% of cases is seen in those over 6 years of age.

20 a) **True**   Polysplenia or bilateral left-sidedness is associated with two morphological left lungs, biliary atresia, absence of the gall bladder, malrotation and cardiovascular abnormalities.

     b) **True**   Seen in 80% of cases.

     c) **False**   Asplenia may have bilateral right-sidedness. There are two morphological right lungs, midline location of the liver, reversed position of the aorta and IVC and total anomalous pulmonary venous drainage is seen in nearly 100% of cases. Other associations include: gastrointestinal anomalies (situs inversus, annular pancreas, Hirschsprung's disease), renal anomalies (horseshoe kidney, duplex system, absent left adrenal gland, bicornuate uterus) and cardiac defects (endocardial cushion defect, single ventricle, dextrocardia).

     d) **False**   See c) above. Genitourinary anomalies are seen in 15% of cases.

     e) **True**   Howell–Jolly bodies in the peripheral blood are a feature of an absent spleen.

Chapter 3

Abdominal imaging

1 **In abdominal lymphoma, which of the following are true?**
   a) Multifocal nodules are the most common pattern of splenic involvement
   b) Splenic involvement is reliably diagnosed with magnetic resonance imaging (MRI)
   c) Liver involvement is seen in 60% of patients with Hodgkin's lymphoma
   d) The small intestine is the most common gastrointestinal site of involvement
   e) The caecum is the most common site of colonic involvement

2 **Which of the following are true regarding trauma to the gastrointestinal tract?**
   a) Acutely clotted blood within the abdomen typically has CT attenuation values of 50–60 Hounsfield units (HU)
   b) The terminal ileum is the most common site of bowel laceration
   c) Jejunal laceration is frequently associated with pneumoperitoneum
   d) Interloop fluid of water density on CT is a useful sign of bowel perforation
   e) A small hypodense spleen is a feature of haemorrhagic shock

3 **Which of the following are true regarding the kidney?**
   a) The presence of cyst calcification in patients with adult polycystic kidney disease confers a high risk of renal malignancy
   b) The ipsilateral adrenal gland is involved in 10% of patients with renal cell carcinoma
   c) In renal cell carcinoma, the demonstration of stranding in the perinephric space on CT indicates tumour extension beyond the kidney
   d) Gradient echo sequences have greater accuracy in the detection of inferior vena cava (IVC) tumour thrombosis than spin echo sequences
   e) Lymphangioleiomyomatosis of the kidney is associated with tuberous sclerosis

4 **Regarding hepatocellular carcinomas, which of the following are true?**
   a) They are commonly hyperechoic on ultrasonography
   b) The majority are hyperdense during the arterial phase on CT
   c) The majority are hyperintense on T1-weighted and T2-weighted imaging
   d) The central scar may be hypointense on T2-weighted imaging
   e) Portal or hepatic venous invasion is seen on MRI in one third of patients

5 **Which of the following are true regarding fibrolamellar hepatocellular carcinoma?**
   a) The majority are associated with elevated alphafetoprotein
   b) A central scar is present in 50% of cases on ultrasonography
   c) Calcification is rarely seen on CT
   d) There is delayed enhancement of the tumour following intravenous gadolinium on MRI
   e) The central scar may enhance following intravenous contrast on CT

6 **Which of the following are true regarding testicular tumours?**
   a) Seminomas are highly radiosensitive
   b) About 90% of nongerm cell tumours are benign
   c) Lymphoma typically presents as a focal hypoechoic mass on ultrasonography
   d) Yolk sac tumours usually spread by lymphatic dissemination
   e) Isolated involvement of the external iliac nodes rarely occurs

7   **In the imaging of acute testicular torsion, which of the following are true?**
   a)   Surgery is successful in 20% of patients who present between 12 and 24 hours after onset of symptoms
   b)   On sonography, a reactive hydrocoele is seen after 6 hours
   c)   Colour Doppler ultrasound may show increased blood flow in the epididymis
   d)   Hyperperfusion of the testicle on colour Doppler ultrasonography makes testicular torsion unlikely
   e)   Technetium-99m pertechnetate scintigraphy typically shows a halo of hyperactivity in the acute phase (first 6 hours)

8   **Which of the following liver lesions may demonstrate signal loss on out-of-phase (opposed phase) MRI?**
   a)   Hepatocellular carcinoma
   b)   Cholangiocarcinoma
   c)   Lymphoma
   d)   Hepatocellular adenoma
   e)   Haemangioma

9   **Which of the following are true of cystic fibrosis?**
   a)   Chronic liver disease is present in 75% of adults with cystic fibrosis
   b)   The most common abdominal MRI finding is fatty infiltration of the pancreas
   c)   Pancreatic calcification is seen in 30% of patients on radiography
   d)   Pancreatic cysts are a common finding
   e)   Microgallbladder is a rare finding

10   **Which of the following are true regarding Behçet's syndrome?**
   a)   The gastrointestinal tract is involved in up to 40% of cases
   b)   The jejunum is the most common site involved within the gastrointestinal tract
   c)   Deep ulceration of the bowel wall is typical
   d)   Pericolonic infiltration is a typical feature on CT in uncomplicated cases
   e)   Necrolytic erythema migrans is an associated finding

11   **In ultrasonography of the renal tract, which of the following are true?**
   a)   Pregnancy-related renal dilatation is present by the tenth week of gestation
   b)   In pregnancy-related dilatation of the collecting system, the right side is involved in most cases
   c)   The resistive index (RI) in intrarenal arteries is normally greater than 0.7
   d)   Renal cancers are rarely hyperechoic at ultrasound
   e)   A hyperechoic lesion with posterior acoustic shadowing in the absence of calcification on ultrasound is more suggestive of angiomyolipoma than renal cell carcinoma

12   **In carcinoma of the oesophagus, which of the following are true?**
   a)   Oesophageal cancer is associated with coeliac disease
   b)   Pericardial effusion suggests unresectability
   c)   Five-year survival in oesophageal cancer patients without nodal disease is 48%
   d)   Barrett's oesophagus is associated with squamous metaplasia of the distal oesophagus
   e)   Endoscopic ultrasonography (EUS) is more accurate than endoscopy in diagnosing recurrent oesophageal cancer

13 Which of the following are true concerning benign lesions of the oesophagus?
 a) Duplication cysts are completely surrounded by muscularis propria
 b) Duplication cysts typically are of water density on CT
 c) Leiomyomas are more common in the proximal oesophagus
 d) Hypertrophic osteoarthropathy may be a feature of leiomyomas
 e) Giant oesophageal ulcer is a feature of cytomegalovirus (CMV) oesophagitis

14 Which of the following are true regarding radiation enteritis?
 a) Enteritis typically develops after a dose of 4 500 cGy
 b) The underlying pathology is endarteritis
 c) Hypertension is a predisposing factor
 d) Effacement of mucosal folds is a typical feature on barium studies
 e) MRI findings are specific

15 In imaging tumours of the small bowel, which of the following are true?
 a) Adenocarcinoma is more common in the distal small bowel than the proximal bowel
 b) Ulceration is a frequent feature of adenocarcinoma
 c) Leiomyomas show marked enhancement on contrast-enhanced CT
 d) Focal aneurysmal dilatations of the bowel are a feature of lymphoma
 e) Thickening of the valvulae conniventes is a typical feature of Mediterranean lymphoma

16 In inflammatory bowel disease, which of the following are true?
 a) Homogenous enhancement of the bowel wall on contrast-enhanced CT is a feature of Crohn's disease
 b) Bowel wall thickening is greater in Crohn's disease than in ulcerative colitis
 c) Fibro-fatty mesenteric proliferation is present in 40% of patients with Crohn's disease
 d) Submucosal fat deposition is a feature of chronic ulcerative colitis
 e) Widening of the presacral space is a feature of ulcerative colitis

17 Which of the following are true regarding mucosal associated lymphoid tissue (MALT) lymphoma of the gastrointestinal tract?
 a) The normal stomach does not contain lymphoid follicles
 b) MALT lymphoma is widely disseminated at the time of diagnosis in most patients
 c) The most common site within the stomach is the antrum
 d) Ulceration is a common feature on barium study
 e) Perforation of the stomach is a recognised feature of gastric MALT lymphoma

18 Which of the following are true regarding imaging of the small bowel?
 a) Loss of haustrations is a typical feature of graft-versus-host disease
 b) Thickening of the valvulae conniventes is a typical feature of Henoch–Schönlein purpura
 c) Marked bowel dilatation is a feature of intestinal lymphangiectasia
 d) Distal small bowel is more commonly involved than proximal small bowel in scleroderma
 e) Duodenal stricture is a feature of *Strongyloides* infection

19 In the imaging of portal hypertension, which of the following are true?

a) Coronary vein collaterals are the most common varices seen on portal venography
b) Oesophageal varices are supplied by the anterior branch of the left gastric vein
c) Para-umbilical varices are present in 75% of patients with portal hypertension
d) Endoscopy is a reliable method of detecting gastric varices
e) Para-oesophageal varices appear as a posterior mediastinal mass on radiography

20 Which of the following are true regarding imaging of liver transplantation?

a) Hepatic artery thrombosis is the most common vascular complication
b) Portal vein thrombosis usually occurs within 24 hours of transplantation
c) Hepatic vein stenosis is more common following living related transplants than after cadaveric transplants
d) Periportal low attenuation on contrast-enhanced CT is a reliable sign of acute graft rejection
e) Biliary anastomotic stenoses are reliably diagnosed using magnetic resonance cholangiopancreatography (MRCP)

21 Regarding focal nodular hyperplasia (FNH), which of the following are true?

a) There is a strong causal association with the oral contraceptive pill
b) Most cases are solitary
c) There is early intense enhancement on contrast-enhanced CT
d) The central scar is seen in more than 70% of cases on MRI
e) The lesion appears hyperintense on MRI following intravenous mangafodipir trisodium

22 In the imaging of the liver, which of the following are true?

a) The hepatic artery lies within the lesser omentum
b) A hypodense rim surrounding a focal lesion is more suggestive of a haemangioma than a metastasis on contrast-enhanced CT
c) Most hepatocellular adenomas have high signal relative to normal liver on T1-weighted MRI
d) Calcification is seen in 10% of hepatocellular carcinomas on CT
e) Hyperintensity on T1-weighted imaging is helpful in differentiating hepatocellular carcinoma from metastasis

23 Which of the following are true regarding the gall bladder?

a) 95% of cases of acute cholecystitis are caused by an obstructing calculus in the cystic duct
b) MRCP has 95% sensitivity for cystic duct stones
c) The most common site of biliary-enteric fistula formation is between the gallbladder fundus and the duodenal bulb
d) Metastases are present in 25% of carcinomas of the gallbladder at presentation
e) Pneumobilia is a common feature of emphysematous cholecystitis

24 Which of the following are true of pancreatic carcinoma?

a) CA 19-9 is elevated in more than 80% of patients with ductal adenocarcinoma
b) Ductal adenocarcinoma has reduced signal on T1-weighted and T2-weighted MRI relative to normal pancreas
c) The loss of a fat plane around the superior mesenteric artery is indicative of invasion
d) Solid and papillary neoplasms are usually locally invasive at diagnosis
e) Intraductal papillary mucinous subtypes are characterised by hyperintense pancreatic ducts on T2-weighted MRI

25 Regarding pancreatic masses, which of the following are true?
a) Pancreatic cysts are seen in 40% of patients with adult polycystic kidney disease
b) There is an association between von Hippel–Lindau syndrome (VHL) and pancreatic ductal adenocarcinoma
c) Serous microcystic neoplasm (serous cystadenoma) is hypervascular at angiography
d) Mucinous cystic neoplasms (cystadenocarcinoma) occur most frequently in the pancreatic head
e) Islet cell tumours commonly show cystic change

26 In the imaging of acute colitis, which of the following are true?
a) Paucity of pericolonic inflammation is more suggestive of pseudomembranous colitis than ulcerative colitis
b) In pseudomembranous colitis, the most common site involved is the rectosigmoid
c) Toxic megacolon is not a feature of pseudomembranous colitis
d) Portal venous gas is a more specific sign of ischaemic colitis than pneumatosis cystoides intestinalis
e) Neutropenic colitis (typhlitic colitis) most commonly affects the descending and sigmoid colon

27 In Whipple's disease, which of the following are true?
a) Females are more commonly affected
b) Sacroiliitis is a feature
c) Small bowel dilatation is a typical finding
d) Ulceration is a common finding on barium studies
e) Involved lymph nodes are hypodense on CT

28 Regarding colorectal cancer, which of the following are true?
a) Radiation colitis is a predisposing factor
b) T3 cancer indicates spread beyond the colonic wall
c) 30% of polyps are not detected by a faecal occult blood test
d) Most recurrent cancers are endoluminal at diagnosis
e) 80% of recurrences present within 2 years

29 In the imaging of rectal carcinoma, which of the following are true?
a) MRI does not demonstrate tumour extension to the circumferential resection margin
b) Reduction in local recurrence is better achieved with postoperative radiotherapy than preoperative radiotherapy
c) Involvement of the submucosal veins on MRI is a poor prognostic sign
d) Recurrent tumour following abdominoperineal resection commonly involves the pyriformis muscle
e) Peritoneal involvement is present in 25% of cases

30 Which of the following are true regarding tissue harmonic imaging on ultrasound?
a) Harmonic waves are generated within body tissues
b) Axial resolution is better than with conventional ultrasonography
c) Artefacts are reduced compared with conventional ultrasonography
d) There is better visualisation of fat and calcium when compared with conventional ultrasound
e) Pulse inversion ultrasound is useful for lesions more than 10 cm in depth

31 Regarding imaging of the spleen, which of the following are true?
a) Melanoma is the most common primary tumour to metastasise to the spleen
b) Splenic cysts are a common finding at ultrasound
c) Pyogenic abscesses of the spleen are usually secondary to penetrating trauma
d) Ultrasound typically shows multiple cystic lesions in splenic haemangiomata
e) Angiosarcoma of the spleen is secondary to thorotrast exposure

32 In the abdominal imaging of HIV seropositive patients, which of the following are true?
a) Cryptosporidiosis is associated with pneumatosis cystoides intestinalis
b) *Mycobacterium avium-intracellulare* complex enteritis is associated with low-density lymphadenopathy
c) CMV colitis usually affects the distal colon
d) Amoebiasis has a predilection for the caecum
e) Kaposi's sarcoma affects the gastrointestinal tract in 5% of cases

33 Which of the following are true of gastric cancer?
a) The majority of early gastric cancers arise in the distal half of the stomach
b) Liver metastases are present in 45% of patients at presentation
c) Gastric cancers typically enhance on CT following intravenous contrast
d) A T3 cancer on EUS indicates invasion of the serosa
e) On CT, ascites indicates the presence of peritoneal disease

34 Which of the following are true regarding phaeochromocytomas?
a) In adults, 90% of cases arise from the adrenal medulla
b) They are markedly hyperintense on T2-weighted MRI
c) About 10% of extra-adrenal phaeochromocytomas are malignant
d) There is typically maximal enhancement on the immediate postgadolinium MRI
e) The normal adrenal medulla is well demonstrated with ^{131}I metaiodobenzylguanidine (MIBG) imaging

35 In recurrent cervical cancer, which of the following are true?
a) Hydronephrosis occurs in 70% of cases
b) Para-aortic nodes are generally involved before pelvic side-wall nodes
c) Liver metastases occur in 30% of cases
d) Adrenal gland involvement is rare
e) The rectum is rarely involved

36 Which of the following are true regarding ovarian cancer?
a) About 75% of ovarian neoplasms are benign
b) Lesions greater than 4 cm on CT are suggestive of malignancy
c) Mediastinal lymph node involvement is a rare finding
d) The liver is the most common site of haematogenous metastasis
e) Serous cystadenocarcinoma contains calcification in 30% of cases on CT

37 In hydatid disease, which of the following are true?
a) The liver is involved in 75% of cases
b) Calcification is seen radiographically in 30% of cases with liver involvement
c) Hepatic hydatid cysts typically have a high signal rim on T2-weighted MRI
d) Rupture of the hepatic cysts occurs in 10% of cases
e) Peritoneal seeding occurs in a large proportion of liver hydatid disease

38 Regarding cholangiocarcinoma, which of the following are true?
a) Caroli's disease is a predisposing factor
b) The majority are squamous cell carcinomas
c) It typically shows delayed enhancement on CT
d) Tumours are low signal relative to liver on T2-weighted MRI
e) Duodenal obstruction is an early feature

39 Regarding carcinoid tumour of the gastrointestinal tract, which of the following are true?
a) The jejunum is the most common site of involvement in the small bowel
b) Metastases from carcinoid of the appendix are rare
c) Low-density lymphadenopathy is a feature on CT
d) One third of patients have a second malignancy
e) Multiple lesions are rare

40 Which of the following are true regarding bladder cancers?
a) Urachal abnormalities are most frequently associated with squamous cell carcinomas
b) MRI can identify muscle invasion
c) Tumour extension to the cervix is common
d) The presence of low signal within the seminal vesicles on T2-weighted MRI
   is specific for tumour involvement
e) Bladder cancer enhances early following intravenous gadolinium-
   diethylenetriaminepentaacetic acid (DTPA)

Answers

1 a) **False** The spleen is involved in 40% of cases at laparotomy. The spleen is usually diffusely involved but splenic size is not a reliable indicator of lymphomatous involvement. Less commonly, there may be nodular involvement of the spleen and liver. The nodules are hypoechoic on ultrasonography, exhibit low attenuation on computed tomography (CT), and are hypo/isointense on T1-weighted and hyperintense on T2-weighted MRI.

   b) **False** The normal and diffusely involved spleen may have a similar appearance on MRI.

   c) **True** The liver is involved in 60% of Hodgkin's lymphoma and 50% of non-Hodgkin's lymphoma at autopsy. Diffuse involvement is much more common than focal disease (10%).

   d) **False** The stomach is the most common site of involvement. The infiltrating form is most common and may be difficult to distinguish from scirrhous carcinoma.

   e) **True** The caecum accounts for 85% of colonic involvement.

2 a) **True** Free lysed blood has an attenuation of 25 HU. The sentinel loop sign indicates the proximity of the anatomical injury to the site with the highest attenuation of free fluid.

   b) **False** The most common site of bowel laceration is where the bowel is fixed at the ligament of Treitz. Jejunal laceration is the most common site of perforation.

   c) **False** The proximal jejunum is usually free of gas, so perforation is not frequently associated with pneumoperitoneum.

   d) **True** Free intraperitoneal fluid (HU less than 15) from small bowel perforation may collect between mesenteric reflections, and water density interloop fluid may be the only sign of small bowel perforation.

   e) **True** Following haemorrhagic shock, there is intense vasoconstriction, which may involve the splenic artery branches. This leads to a small homogenously hypoattenuating spleen. Other signs of hypovolaemic shock include flattened IVC, small aorta and mesenteric arteries, lack of renal contrast excretion, marked enhancement of the adrenal glands and generalised thickening and dilatation of the small bowel folds with luminal fluid due to mesenteric vessel vasoconstriction.

3 a) **False** The presence of cyst calcification in patients with this autosomal dominant condition carries less risk of malignancy than it does with cyst calcification in the general population.

   b) **True** The contralateral gland is rarely involved.

   c) **False** Thickening of renal fascia, stranding and tortuous vessels in the perinephric space on CT are poor predictors of tumour extension. They are frequently secondary to oedema, inflammation or engorgement of vessels from increased tumour blood flow. The distinction between stage I (confined disease) and stage II (extension into the perinephric fat) may not be important as both are treated by nephrectomy and have a favourable prognosis.

   d) **True** Extension into the IVC indicates stage III disease. This is seen with tumours larger than 4.5 cm. Signs include distension of the vein, filling defects within the contrast opacified lumen or vessel occlusion with paravertebral collaterals. On CT imaging, the tumour may be isodense with venous blood and may be missed. MRI is more accurate in assessing venous invasion than CT and may be equal to venography. Tumour thrombus replaces the normal signal void on spin echo imaging, but slow flowing blood may also give this appearance. On gradient echo sequences, the thrombus appears as a low-signal filling defect against the high signal flowing blood.

   e) **True** Lymphangioleiomyomatosis results from smooth muscle proliferation that obstructs the lymphatic vessels, resulting in cysts. The most common site is the thorax. Other associations of the condition include angiomyolipomas of the kidney (40%–80%), renal cysts (15%) and renal cell cancer (1%). Renal failure rarely occurs.

4 a) **False** The ultrasonographic appearance is variable. Small tumours are usually uniformly hypoechoic. Large tumours are of mixed echogenicity. Rarely, the tumours may be very echogenic due to fat and resemble haemangiomas. Other features include: hypoechoic rim, target appearance with a hypoechoic halo, mosaic pattern and lateral shadowing. Continuous or pulsatile flow within the lesion on Doppler ultrasonography is also suspicious.

   b) **True** They are hypodense on unenhanced CT. Focal calcification is rarely seen. The majority are hyperattenuating during the arterial phase following intravenous contrast, but 10% are hypoattenuating. Venous invasion is seen in up to 48% on CT. Other features include: thick tumour capsule due to compressed liver tissue, hypodense central scar that does not enhance, fatty change and arterio-portal shunting seen as early and prolonged portal vein enhancement.

   c) **False** On MRI, most are hypointense on T1-weighted and hyperintense on T2-weighted imaging (54% of patients). Other MRI appearances include: isointensity on T1-weighted and T2-weighted imaging (16%), hypointensity on T1-weighted and isointensity on T2-weighted imaging (10%) and hyperintensity on T1-weighted and T2-weighted imaging (6%). Following intravenous gadolinium contrast, there is early enhancement during the arterial phase.

   d) **True** The central scar is hypointense on T1-weighted imaging and may be hypointense or hyperintense on T2-weighted imaging.

   e) **True** Portal or venous invasion is seen in one third of cases on MRI.

5 a) **False** Fibrolamellar carcinoma is not associated with chronic liver disease and tumour markers are not usually elevated. Elevated neurotensin and vitamin B_{12} binding capacity have been reported.

b) **True** The ultrasonographic appearances are variable. The central scar is seen as hyperechoic lines.

c) **False** Calcification is present in 40% of cases on CT. The tumours are usually large (mean size 12 cm), hypodense on unenhanced CT and hyperdense during the arterial phase following intravenous contrast.

d) **False** On MRI, these tumours are heterogeneously hypointense on T1-weighted imaging and hyperintense on T2-weighted imaging. Following gadolinium contrast, the tumour enhances heterogeneously during the arterial phase.

e) **True** The central scar may show delayed enhancement on MRI and CT.

6 a) **True** Germ cell tumours can be divided into seminomas and nonseminomatous types. Seminomas are highly radiosensitive and advanced disease is treated by radiation (although chemotherapy is used increasingly). Advanced nonseminomatous tumours are treated with lymphadenectomy and/or chemotherapy. The primary tumour in both types is treated with orchidectomy.

b) **True** Nongerm cell tumours of the testes arise from Leydig's and Sertoli's cells or the connective tissue stroma and are benign in 90% of cases.

c) **False** Lymphoma usually presents as a homogeneous, hypoechoic mass, which diffusely replaces the testes. The tunica vaginalis is usually intact and the tumour may be demonstrated extending into the epididymis and spermatic cord. Lymphoma is usually of the non-Hodgkin's type and is the most common primary tumour of the testes in those over the age of 60 years.

d) **False** Most testicular tumours spread by lymphatic dissemination, but choriocarcinoma and yolk sac carcinoma spread haematogenously.

e) **True** The lymphatic drainage of the testes is predominantly to the lymph nodes near the renal hilum. After involvement of the sentinel renal hilar nodes, spread occurs to the para-aortic nodes. Subsequent spread to the mediastinal nodes or haematogenous dissemination can occur. Both testes may also drain to the external iliac nodes, but this is more common after primary drainage has been disrupted by surgery at the groin.

7 a) **True** The success of surgical intervention is dependent upon the time from the onset of symptoms to the time of surgery. Surgery is almost 100% successful within 6 hours of onset of symptoms. After 24 hours, the testicle is beyond salvage and must be removed. The infarcted testis can have detrimental effects on the contralateral testis due to the formation of autoantibodies.

b) **True** The appearances are usually normal for the first 4 hours. Between 4 and 6 hours, the testis is enlarged and appears hypoechoic. Later, there is haemorrhage, oedema and ischaemia and the testis is heterogeneous and echogenic. If it is not removed, the testis involutes and becomes small and hypoechoic.

c) **True** Rarely, the testis may tort independently of the epididymis, due to a long mesorchium. In such a case, the epididymis shows reactive hyperaemia.

d) **False** Spontaneous detorsion may occur leading to unilateral testicular hyperperfusion. Surgery is still indicated in these cases.

e) **False** Scintigraphy is highly sensitive and specific when performed early. In the acute phase, there is reduced perfusion in the testis with decreased activity. In the subacute phase (6–15 hours), there is peritesticular reactive hyperaemia with a halo of increased tracer activity. Later, there is marked absence of tracer activity.

8 a) **True**
b) **False**
c) **False**
d) **True**
e) **False**

Loss of signal on opposed phase MRI indicates intracellular lipid and steatosis. Fatty infiltration occurs in 14% of hepatocellular carcinomas and 68% of adenomas, which may result in T1-weighted hyperintensity. Rarely, focal nodular hyperplasia may also demonstrate signal loss on opposed phase MRI.

9 a) **False** Chronic liver disease is present in 25% of adults with cystic fibrosis and the severity increases with age.

b) **True** The most common MRI findings are lobulated fatty replacement of the pancreas, atrophy with partial fatty replacement and diffuse atrophy without fatty replacement.

c) **False** Pancreatic calcification is seen in 8% of patients on radiography. MRI depicts the calcification poorly.

d) **True** Pancreatic cysts are usually small and well depicted on MRI.

e) **False** Microgallbladder is a common finding (seen in 20%–50% of cystic fibrosis cases at autopsy). In patients with cystic fibrosis, the gallbladder is typically small, trabeculated, contracted and poorly functioning. It often contains echogenic bile, sludge and cholesterol gallstones. These changes are due to the thick tenacious bile that is characteristic of this disease.

10 a) **True** The gastrointestinal tract is involved in 10%–40% of cases of Behçet's syndrome. Major criteria include buccal/genital ulceration, ocular lesions, such as iridocyclitis, and dermal lesions. The terminal ileum is the most common site in gastrointestinal involvement.

   b) **False** See a).

   c) **True** Ulcers are deep and hence complications include: perforation, haemorrhage, fistula and peritonitis.

   d) **False** CT features of bowel involvement include concentric wall thickening with marked enhancement. In the absence of complications such as perforation, pericolonic or peri-enteric inflammatory changes are minimal.

   e) **False** Associated features include: erythema nodosum, migratory thrombophlebitis, chronic meningoencephalitis and retinal vasculitis. Necrolytic erythema migrans is seen in glucagonomas.

11 a) **True** Dilatation begins at 10 weeks' gestation. This may be related to relaxation of the distal ureter secondary to raised progesterone levels.

   b) **True** The right side is affected in 85% of cases.

   c) **False** The normal RI is less than 0.7. In pregnancy this does not change significantly. In acute ureteric obstruction the RI rises above 0.7 and may decrease soon after resolution of the obstruction. Ureteric obstruction in pregnancy can be difficult to distinguish from pregnancy-related renal dilatation. Features to suggest the former include marked dilatation (grade III), extension of a dilated ureter across the common iliac artery (as opposed to tapering of the ureter in pregnancy-related dilatation), raised RI and absence of ureteric jets.

   d) **False** About 30% of small renal cancers may be hyperechoic resembling angiomyolipoma. These lesions should be investigated with CT to confirm the presence of fat.

   e) **True** However, this is seen in only 21% of angiomyolipomas. Renal cancer is more likely to have cystic areas or a hypoechoic rim than the pattern described.

12 a) **True** Other associations include hereditary tylosis, Barrett's oesophagus, smoking, Plummer–Vinson syndrome and ethanol abuse.

   b) **True** Other features suggesting unresectability include: intraluminal mass in airway, tumour extension between trachea and aortic arch or between left main bronchus and descending aorta, more than 90 degrees' contact with the aortic circumference, pleural thickening or effusion adjacent to the tumour, and nodal involvement in the mediastinum or coeliac axis.

   c) **True** The 5-year survival with nodal disease is 6%–15%. Nodal involvement is a poor prognostic factor.

   d) **False** Barrett's oesophagus is associated with columnar metaplasia due to chronic reflux oesophagitis; hence, there is increased incidence of adenocarcinoma. These tumours occur in the distal oesophagus and have a tendency to invade the gastric fundus.

   e) **True** EUS is also more accurate than CT in the local staging of oesophageal cancer and is particularly useful for tumours confined to the mucosa and submucosa. Local nodes may be sampled at EUS. Recurrent cancer is also usefully evaluated at EUS. Positron emission tomography has an increasing role in detecting recurrence.

13 a) **True** Duplication cysts appearing as intramural masses and on barium study are indistinguishable from other mural masses, such as leiomyoma.

  b) **True** Duplication cysts have a fluid density and are usually low signal on T1-weighted imaging and high signal on T2-weighted imaging. However, increasing protein may result in high signal on T1-weighted imaging.

  c) **False** Leiomyomas are benign tumours of smooth muscle and are, therefore, more common in the distal rather than the proximal oesophagus. They arise from all layers of the wall (shown well with EUS) and appear as homogenously enhancing, well-defined masses on CT. Multiple leiomyomas may be associated with congenital neural deafness and renal impairment (Alport's syndrome).

  d) **True** However, hypertrophic osteoarthropathy is rare.

  e) **True** However, HIV is a more common cause of giant oesophageal ulceration than CMV.

14 a) **True** Radiation enteritis is an obliterative endarteritis following doses in excess of 4,500 cGy.

  b) **True** See a).

  c) **True** Other factors that impair the microcirculation (such as diabetes mellitus, atherosclerosis, adhesions and prior peritonitis) also predispose to radiation enteritis.

  d) **True** Other features include: thickening of the valvulae conniventes, ulceration, stenosis, fistula and sinus tract formation.

  e) **False** CT and MRI show nonspecific bowel wall thickening and increased mesenteric vascular markings.

15 a) **False** Adenocarcinoma is usually solitary and located in the proximal small bowel.

  b) **True** Other features include annular constriction with shouldering, marked desmoplastic reaction or polyps.

  c) **True** Leiomyomas are more common in the jejunum and ileum (80% of cases) than elsewhere in the small bowel and are usually solitary. On CT, they are smooth and well defined and show uniform or rim enhancement.

  d) **True** Lymphoma of the small bowel is more common distally and may present as a large cavitating, ulcerating or nodular mass with aneurysmal dilatation of the bowel lumen.

  e) **True** Thickening of the valvulae conniventes is uncommon and is typically seen with familial Mediterranean lymphoma.

16 a) **True** In ulcerative colitis, inhomogeneous mural wall enhancement is seen in 70% on contrast-enhanced CT. The mural heterogeneity is thought to be due to submucosal fat deposition, which is seen in the subacute and chronic phase.

  b) **True** CT demonstrates homogenous thickening of the bowel wall.

  c) **True** Fibro-fatty proliferation is seen in 40% of patients with Crohn's disease and is a common cause of bowel loop separation.

  d) **True** See a).

  e) **True** Other features may include narrowing of the rectum, rectal wall thickening and perirectal fat stranding. The normal presacral space measures less than 5 mm in 95% of patients. A presacral space greater than 10 mm is definitely abnormal. Other causes of widened presacral space include proctitis, carcinoma, haematoma, sacral tumour and congenital lesions, such as rectal duplication cysts.

17 a) **True** However, lymphoid follicles can develop following infection with *Helicobacter pylori*. The acquired lymphoid tissue is of the MALT type. Persistent antigenic stimulation by *H. pylori* is thought to lead to neoplastic transformation.

b) **False** In addition, MALT lymphoma generally has a better prognosis than non-Hodgkin's lymphoma.

c) **True** The most common site of *H. pylori* infection is the gastric antrum. See a).

d) **False** The most common pattern on barium study is infiltrative, either focal or diffuse. Ulcerative lesions, especially in the stomach, are rare.

e) **True** Perforation is a recognised but uncommon finding.

18 a) **True** Other features on barium study include: effacement of the small bowel with a tubular appearance, fold thickening, persistent coating of the bowel mucosa by barium and markedly decreased transit time.

b) **True** Henoch–Schönlein purpura is an allergic vasculitis characterised by a purpuric rash, glomerulonephritis with microscopic haematuria, arthralgia and abdominal pain. Haemorrhage and oedema produce thickening of the valvulae conniventes.

c) **False** Intestinal lymphangiectasia involves dilatation of the lymphatics and may be primary (associated with atresia of the thoracic duct) or secondary (associated with retroperitoneal fibrosis, pancreatitis, diffuse small bowel lymphoma and mesenteric adenitis). It is characterised by a protein-losing enteropathy and barium studies show diffuse symmetrical thickening of the duodenal and jejunal folds, dilution of barium and little or no bowel dilatation.

d) **False** The small bowel is involved in 45% of cases of scleroderma. Proximal bowel dilatation, especially of the duodenum (megaduodenum), is a typical feature. Other features on barium study include a hidebound pattern in 60% of cases (decreased intervalvular distance with well-defined folds of normal thickness), pseudodiverticula, pneumatosis cystoides intestinalis and a prolonged transit time.

e) **True** *Strongyloides stercoralis* is a helminthic parasite, which traverses the lungs and reaches the duodenum and jejunum, where it causes oedema and inflammation due to invasion by the developing larvae. Fold thickening, stenosis of the third and fourth parts of the duodenum, and dilatation of the more proximal duodenum are all recognised findings.

19 a) **True** Coronary vein collaterals (dilated left gastric vein greater than 6 mm) are seen in 86% of cases of portal hypertension on angiography and 80% on dynamic contrast CT. They are seen within the gastro–hepatic ligament. Ultrasound usually identifies the caudal segment near the portal vein and CT identifies the cephalic segment near the gastro-oesophageal junction. They are usually associated with oesophageal and para-oesophageal varices.

b) **True** Oesophageal varices are dilated mucosal and submucosal veins, which are usually supplied by the anterior branch of the left gastric vein. The posterior branch usually supplies the para-oesophageal varices. On CT, they appear as scalloped, enhancing areas of thickening in the lower oesophageal wall with intraluminal projections.

c) **False** Para-umbilical venous collaterals are seen in up to 30% of patients with portal hypertension. They are supplied by the left portal vein and lie in the falciform ligament. CT is more sensitive than angiography in detecting their presence.

d) **False** Endoscopy and barium studies are limited in the diagnosis of gastric varices, which lie deep within the mucosa or serosa. Portal venography and CT are equally sensitive in their detection.

e) **True** Para-oesophageal varices lie in the posterior mediastinum and in 8% of cases can appear as a posterior mediastinal mass on radiography.

20 a) **True** Hepatic artery thrombosis may lead to a biliary leak, stricture and hepatic infarction, and is more common in paediatric liver transplantation. Thrombosis can be confidently diagnosed on Doppler ultrasonography, and hepatic infarction on contrast-enhanced CT.

b) **False** Portal vein stenosis or thrombosis develops slowly, presenting with varices, splenomegaly and ascites. Portal vein stenosis may be treated by balloon dilatation, but once the thrombus is extensive and reaches the periphery of the intrahepatic portal vein branches, then repeat liver transplant is the only alternative.

c) **True** In living related transplant, the hepatic vein is reconstructed without the IVC by end-to-end or end-to-side anastomosis. Anastomotic stenoses may result.

d) **False** Although periportal low attenuation on contrast-enhanced CT may be a feature of acute graft rejection, it has poor sensitivity and specificity and is frequently seen with oedema of the periportal lymphatic vessels.

e) **False** Ultrasonography, CT and MRCP are not as reliable as percutaneous transhepatic cholangiography in the diagnosis of anastomotic strictures. Biliary strictures are seen in 20% of cases and are most common in children following live, related donor transplantation.

21 a) **False** It is generally agreed that oral contraceptive pills do not cause FNH, but discontinuation of these can result in reduction in the size of the lesion. Oestrogen is thought to have a trophic effect.

b) **True** About 80% of cases of FNH are solitary and usually subcapsular.

c) **True** After contrast, there is intense enhancement during the arterial phase. The lesion becomes isointense during the portal venous phase. The sensitivity of CT in detecting the lesion is 78%.

d) **True** The central scar is seen in 20% of cases on ultrasound, 60% on contrast-enhanced CT and 78% on MRI. On MRI, FNH is isointense or slightly hypointense on T1-weighted imaging and slightly hyperintense on T2-weighted imaging. During the arterial phase following intravenous gadolinium, FNH is hyperintense with a hypointense central scar on T1-weighted imaging. During portal venous phase, the lesion is isointense or slightly hyperintense with a hyperintense central scar on T1-weighted imaging. The central scar is hyperintense on T2-weighted MRI.

e) **True** With hepatobiliary specific contrast, such as mangafodipir trisodium, FNH is hyperintense on T1-weighted imaging with a hypointense central scar.

22 a) **True** The hepatic artery arises from the coeliac axis and enters the lesser omentum. It gives off the right gastric and gastroduodenal branches and travels within the hepatoduodenal ligament to reach the porta hepatis.

b) **False** Haemangiomas typically show peripheral nodular enhancement with progressive centripetal fill-in, although a central non-enhancing fibrotic scar is common in larger lesions. Hypervascular metastases also show early enhancement. However, the density of hypervascular neoplasms often fades more rapidly than adjacent normal vessels and a hypodense rim may be seen, a feature not observed in haemangiomas.

c) **True** Most hepatocellular adenomas are high signal on T1-weighted images due to the presence of fat and haemorrhage. On T2-weighted imaging, they are usually isointense or slightly hyperintense. They enhance following intravenous gadolinium. The MRI appearances are frequently not specific enough to make a confident diagnosis.

d) **True** Most are hypodense on unenhanced CT. After contrast, they are hyperdense during the arterial phase and become iso/hypodense during the portal venous phase.

e) **True** T1-weighted imaging hyperintensity may be present in hepatocellular carcinoma due to the presence of haemorrhage, fatty metamorphosis, copper deposition, or glycogen. Metastases usually return a low T1-weighted image signal. However, benign masses such as adenoma and angiomyolipoma can return a high T1-weighted imaging signal.

23 a) **True** In 80%–95% of cases, the level of obstruction is at the cystic duct.

b) **True** MRCP has a very high sensitivity for cystic duct stones. These appear as low signal filling defects within a high signal bile-filled gallbladder or cystic duct.

c) **False** About 80% of cases of biliary-enteric fistula formation occur between the cystic duct and the duodenum just distal to the bulb. In these cases, the gallbladder is frequently shrunken mimicking a duodenal diverticulum.

d) **False** The tumour is locally advanced at presentation (75% are unresectable) and metastases are present in 75% of cases.

e) **False** Pneumobilia is a rare feature. Characteristic features include air within the gallbladder wall or an air-fluid level within the lumen. About 80% of cases are associated with gallstones and the causative organisms include *Clostridium perfringens/welchii*, *Escherichia coli* and *Staphylococcus*.

24 a) **True** CA 19-9 is elevated in 89% of cases. It is also elevated in 29% of extrapancreatic malignancy and 13% of benign pancreatic disease. Pancreatic carcinoma is also associated with raised alkaline phosphatase (85%), lactate dehydrogenase (69%), bilirubin (55%) and glutamic oxaloacetic transaminase (67%).

b) **True** Tumours are often isodense on unenhanced CT and hypodense relative to enhancing pancreas on the pancreatic phase of enhancement. On MRI, tumours are often hypointense on T1-weighted and T2-weighted imaging. Fat suppression and intravenous gadolinium may increase tumour conspicuity.

c) **True** However, this is less reliable at the splenic/superior mesenteric vein confluence and around the proximal portal vein.

d) **False** These are large (10 cm) tumours that are well demarcated, thick walled (hence less likely to invade locally) and have solid and cystic areas. Imaging shows enhancement of the thick wall with nodular projections from the inner wall margin. They are more common in the body and tail of the pancreas. Calcification may be seen at the periphery. Prognosis is good with a 95% cure rate.

e) **True** These are rare tumours characterised by a dilated pancreatic duct with mucin spilling from the ampulla at endoscopy. They are classified according to location: main duct or branch duct. On MRI, mucin-laden dilated ducts have high signal on T2-weighted imaging and variable signal on T1-weighted imaging.

25 a) **False** Cysts are seen in 10% of patients with adult polycystic kidney disease. The cysts are usually small and may be localised or diffuse. Rarely, pancreatic cysts are the dominant feature.

b) **True** VHL is inherited as an autosomal dominant trait. Clinical manifestations include haemangioblastomas of the central nervous system, retinal angiomas and cystic disease of the liver, kidneys and pancreas. There is an association with epididymal cysts, phaeochromocytomas, pancreatic serous neoplasms, ductal adenocarcinomas and islet cell tumours.

c) **True** Serous microcystic neoplasm is benign and occurs in the elderly with a slight propensity for the pancreatic head. They are usually large and lobulated with a central calcified scar. Multiple small (less than 2 cm) cysts are seen. Their rich capillary network predisposes to haemorrhage.

d) **False** Mucinous cystic neoplasms usually occur within the tail or body (75%) of the pancreas and are more common in females (80%), occurring in the sixth decade. The lesion appears as a unilocular or multilocular hypovascular mass on CT with a thick wall and papillary excrescences, although the septae and wall may enhance after intravenous contrast. The appearance of the cyst varies on MRI, depending on the presence of mucin, haemorrhage and protein content.

e) **False** Islet cell tumours are typically hypervascular lesions. They are usually solid and cystic change is only seen in 10% of cases.

26 a) **True** Pseudomembranous colitis is caused by *Clostridium difficile* enterotoxin. CT features are nonspecific and include mural thickening with bowel dilatation.

b) **False** The disease distribution of pseudomembranous colitis includes: pancolitis (50%), right-sided colitis (27%) and isolated rectosigmoid disease (12%). The rectosigmoid is spared in up to 67% of cases and ascites is not uncommon.

c) **False** Complications of pseudomembranous colitis include toxic megacolon, perforation and peritonitis.

d) **True** The presence of mesenteric vascular thrombosis and portal vein gas strongly suggests ischaemic colitis. Less specific signs include mural wall thickening, mural enhancement, pneumatosis, mesenteric fluid, oedema and haemorrhage. Bowel involvement is often segmental in a vascular territory.

e) **False** Neutropenic colitis is seen in neutropenic patients and usually presents as non-specific thickening of the caecal and ascending colonic wall due to necrosis. Pericolonic inflammation, ascites and pneumatosis are also features.

27 a) **False** Males are more commonly affected (9:1 M:F). Whipple's disease is a systemic disease characterised by intestinal lipodystrophy.

b) **True** Typical features include: migratory arthralgia/arthritis, malabsorption, generalised lymphadenopathy, skin pigmentation, splenomegaly and pleuropericarditis.

c) **False** Barium findings include absence of (or minimal) bowel dilatation, no ulceration and thickening of the duodenal and jejunal folds due to infiltration by periodic acid-Schiff positive glycoprotein containing macrophages.

d) **False** See c).

e) **True** CT shows bulky hypodense abdominal lymph nodes. This appearance may also be observed in patients with AIDS who have *Mycobacterium avium-intracellulare* complex infection (pseudo-Whipple's).

28 a) **True**   Other factors include adenomatous polyps, familial polyposis, ulcerative colitis (pancolitis and duration of disease greater than 10 years) and ureterosigmoidostomy. Additional associations include family history of colorectal carcinoma, history of endometrial or breast cancer, and hereditary nonpolyposis colorectal cancer syndrome (Lynch syndrome).

    b) **True**   T4 indicates spread to neighbouring tissues.

    c) **True**   Additionally, colonoscopy may miss up to 24% of colonic polyps. Flexible sigmoidoscopy fails to evaluate the proximal colon where 45% of colorectal cancers are found.

    d) **False**   5% of recurrent cancers are endoluminal and 50% are extraluminal. Thus, cross-sectional imaging is an important method of follow-up of these patients.

    e) **True**   50% of recurrences present within 1 year and 60% of these recur locally at the anastomosis site. Twenty-six percent recur with distant metastases.

29 a) **False**   The mesorectum on MRI is represented by a hypointense line surrounding the rectum, perirectal fat, blood vessels, lymphatics and nerves. The mesorectum is cleaved along its plane at surgery (total mesorectal excision) with removal *en bloc* of the perirectal lymphatics. This reduces local recurrences of rectal carcinoma and also spares the hypogastric nerves. Tumour deposit that compromises the circumferential resection margin has a high risk of local recurrence. MRI is useful in demonstrating tumour encroaching the circumferential resection margin.

    b) **False**   Preoperative radiotherapy reduces local recurrences significantly, particularly when the circumferential resection margin is compromised.

    c) **False**   Independent poor prognostic factors include: involvement of circumferential resection margins, node positivity, tumour involvement of the extramural veins and peritoneal infiltration.

    d) **True**   Recurrent tumour is usually seen as a homogenous soft tissue mass sometimes with a low-density centre containing gas. It commonly invades the coccygeus and pyriformis muscles. The sciatic nerves may also be involved causing leg pain.

    e) **True**   Local peritoneal spread is a poor independent prognostic sign and may predict recurrence in upper rectal tumours.

30 a) **True**   Harmonic waves are created within body tissues when these tissues are resonated by a specific frequency of transmitted ultrasound. Harmonic waves are made up of frequencies of multiples of the transmitted frequency. Once the transmitted frequency is filtered the image is formed by detecting these harmonic waves.

    b) **True**   This is due to the shorter wavelengths of the harmonic waves and the use of higher effective transmitting frequency. Also, improved focusing due to a higher transmitted frequency allows a narrow beam. This allows better axial resolution.

    c) **True**   The harmonic waves are of low amplitude and scattered waves are less likely to be detected. Harmonic waves are produced within tissues and not at the body surface, which reduces defocusing at the body surface.

    d) **True**   There is better visualisation of lesions containing fat, calcium and air. The technique is particularly useful in obese patients and in patients with cystic lesions; it helps to distinguish cystic lesions from other hypoechoic masses.

    e) **False**   Conventional and harmonic ultrasounds rely on a single pulse of ultrasound. Pulse inversion produces two or more identical ultrasonographic pulses with reversed polarity. This technique produces better image resolution. However, due to attenuation, it is not useful for structures greater than 10 cm in depth.

31 a) **True**   Splenic metastases are seen in 7% of patients with disseminated malignancy. Half of the cases are due to melanoma and the remaining 50% are due to breast, bronchogenic, colonic, renal, ovary and endometrial cancer.

    b) **False**   True splenic cysts (congenital cysts or epidermoid cysts) are an unusual finding within the spleen. Most cysts (80%) are post-traumatic.

    c) **False**   Pyogenic abscesses are secondary to haematogenous dissemination (75%), penetrating trauma (15%) and splenic infarction (10%).

    d) **True**   Multiple cystic lesions within an echogenic mass are seen in splenic haemangiomata. CT shows low attenuation masses resembling cysts with enhancement of the more solid elements following contrast.

    e) **False**   Unlike angiosarcomas of the spleen, angiosarcomas of the liver are secondary to previous thorotrast or polyvinyl chloride exposure. These are rare tumours.

32 a) **True**   Other causes of pneumatosis cystoides intestinalis include: intestinal trauma, ischaemia, peptic ulcer, inflammatory bowel disease, collagen vascular disease, chronic airway disease, asthma and cystic fibrosis.

b) **True**   Other features of *Mycobacterium avium-intracellulare* complex enteritis include: mild dilatation of the mid and distal small bowel, irregular fold thickening and splenomegaly with focal low attenuation lesions in the liver and spleen.

c) **False**   CMV colitis results in a small vessel vasculitis with ischaemic necrosis. The terminal ileum is the most common site of involvement. There may be aphthous ulcers on a background of normal or nodular mucosa. Other features include: marked colonic wall thickening, ascites, toxic megacolon and pericolonic inflammatory changes.

d) **True**   Amoebiasis is caused by *Entamoeba histolytica*. The protozoa invade the mucosa and submucosa causing ulceration and necrosis, with a predilection for the ascending colon and caecum (90% of cases). Radiographic features include: loss of haustra, collarbutton ulcers, scarred cone-shaped colon and stenosis of the bowel lumen. The ileocaecal valve may be thickened and fixed.

e) **True**   About 30% of patients with AIDS develop Kaposi's sarcoma. The skin is the most common site and lesions may encompass the entire gastrointestinal tract. The gastrointestinal tract is the sole site of Kaposi's sarcoma in 5% of cases.

33 a) **True**   Most early cancers are found in the distal half of the stomach, usually along the lesser curve. More recently, there has been an increase in incidence of cancers in the proximal third of the stomach and distal oesophagus.

b) **False**   With advanced gastric cancer, liver metastases are present in 25% of cases. Increasing submucosal spread increases lymph node involvement.

c) **True**   Contrast-enhanced CT usually shows focal or more diffuse enhancing mass involving the gastric wall. More advanced cancer may show transmural enhancement. The accuracy of CT in detection of advanced gastric cancer (T3/T4) is 78%. CT is less accurate for early cancer (T1 and T2).

d) **True**   EUS is more accurate in local (T) staging that CT. Most tumours are seen as hypoechoic lesions with irregular margins. The tumour may be limited to the mucosa and submucosa (T1), limited to the muscularis propria (T2), show serosal invasion (T3) or invade adjacent organs (T4). EUS is more accurate than CT in local staging (staging accuracy 92%). The accuracy of nodal staging is 83%. The limited field of view reduces detection of involved nodes distant from the tumour.

e) **True**   The presence of ascites on CT indicates peritoneal spread. Although discrete peritoneal nodules may not be realised on CT, laparoscopy may detect these lesions earlier. Peritoneal spread is present in 25% of patients at diagnosis.

34 a) **True** The most common location of an extra-adrenal phaeochromocytoma is the aortic bifurcation. Extra-adrenal tumours are more common in children, accounting for 30% of cases.

b) **True** However, this appearance is not diagnostic as adrenal cysts and carcinoma may have a similar, but less hyperintense, appearance.

c) **False** About 40% of extra-adrenal phaeochromocytomas are malignant. About 10% of adrenal phaeochromocytomas are malignant and 10% are bilateral.

d) **False** These tumours usually exhibit greatest enhancement during the later interstitial phase. There is usually mild early enhancement due to few feeding vessels and greater enhancement later due to the large extracellular space.

e) **False** ^{131}I MIBG is an analogue of guanethidine and is taken up actively by the amine transport system. The normal adrenal medulla is either not seen or only faintly demonstrated. Adrenal medullary hyperplasia, phaeochromocytoma, neuroblastoma, ganglioneuroblastoma and paraganglioma show increased uptake of the tracer.

35 a) **True** At autopsy, hydronephrosis occurs in 70% of cases. Local recurrence can also involve the bladder and lead to a vesicovaginal fistula.

b) **False** The paracervical, parametrial, obturator and iliac nodes are involved first. Later there is spread to the common iliac and para-aortic nodes with a progressively worse prognosis.

c) **True** The liver is the most common site of haematogenous metastasis (33%). The adrenal gland is the next most common solid organ to be involved (16%). The kidneys and pancreas may be involved, but this is rare.

d) **False** See c).

e) **False** Recurrent tumours commonly involve the rectum, and rectovaginal fistulae may develop in 17% of cases. Other sites of spread include the peritoneum and chest, where lung metastases and less commonly pleural deposits, endobronchial lesions or pericardial disease may be seen.

36 a) **True** Tumours may arise from the surface epithelium, germ cells or specialised gonadal stroma, but 75% are benign. Malignant tumours account for 21% of cases (borderline type 4%). About 85% of malignant tumours are of the epithelial type.

b) **True** Other features suggestive of malignancy include papillary projections, septa of more than 3 mm and complex cysts with increasingly solid elements and enhancing tumour vessels.

c) **False** Lymph node spread is typically along the path of the gonadal vessels to the para-aortic nodes and along the parametrial channels to the external iliac and hypogastric group. Enlarged paracardiac nodes may be seen in 28% of stage III and recurrent epithelial ovarian cancer. Mediastinal nodal involvement may be seen in up to one third of cases at autopsy.

d) **True** Other sites of haematogenous metastasis include adrenal glands, bone, spleen, pancreas and kidneys.

e) **True** CT may also show calcification within peritoneal nodules and lymph nodes.

37 a) **True** *Echinococcus granulosus* reaches the liver via the portal circulation. The lung is involved in 15% of cases. In the liver, the right lobe is the most frequently involved.

b) **True** Calcification is usually ring-like due to calcification of the pericyst. Complete calcification of the pericyst is seen with its death.

c) **False** On T2-weighted MRI, the cysts have a low signal rim (due to high collagen content). On CT, the cyst walls have high attenuation even in the absence of calcification.

d) **False** Cyst rupture occurs in 50%–90% of cases and can be clinically insidious or lead to anaphylaxis. Rupture may be contained, communicating with the biliary system, or cause free spill into the pleural/peritoneal cavity or hollow viscera when rupture is direct.

e) **False** Peritoneal spread occurs in 13% of cases and is frequently seen after previous surgery. It is typically clinically silent until cysts are large enough to produce symptoms.

38 a) **True** Caroli's disease is characterised by the presence of multiple intrahepatic bile duct cysts, due to cavernous ectasia of the biliary tract, in the absence of liver cirrhosis and portal hypertension. It is associated with renal cysts. Other predisposing factors for cholangiocarcinoma include choledochal cysts, primary sclerosing cholangitis, *Clonorchis sinensis* infection and ulcerative colitis.

b) **False** About 95% of cholangiocarcinomas are adenocarcinomas. Other tumours are rare and include squamous cell carcinoma, lymphoma, carcinoid and mucin-secreting papillary adenocarcinoma.

c) **True** The tumours are generally hypovascular with fibrotic centres and viable cells at the periphery. After intravenous contrast, there is little initial tumour enhancement or only mild rim enhancement. On delayed images, there may be more diffuse and persistent enhancement. The tumour is usually isodense to liver on unenhanced CT.

d) **False** The tumours have varied appearance on T2-weighted imaging, from very high signal to mildly increased signal relative to the liver, depending on the degree of the fibrotic component. On T1-weighting, they are isointense or low signal relative to the liver. After intravenous gadolinium administration, there is moderate enhancement on T1-weighted imaging with better delineation of the tumour than with contrast-enhanced CT.

e) **False** The tumour spreads by local invasion and may involve the portal vein and hepatic artery. Lymphatic spread may also involve the periductal, peripancreatic, and peri-aortic nodes. Duodenal and gastric obstructions are late features.

39 a) **False** Carcinoid is the most common primary malignant tumour of the small bowel. It arises from neuroendocrine cells of the submucosa and may secrete a variety of products (for example: 5-hydroxyindoleacetic acid, adrenocorticoptrophic hormone, histamine and serotonin). A third occur in the small bowel (91% in the ileum, 7% in the jejunum and 2% in the duodenum) and 45% arise in the appendix. Gastric carcinoids are rare.

b) **True** The incidence of metastases, which are usually to the liver and lymph nodes (also lung and bone), is related to tumour size (2% of tumours less than 1 cm metastasise and 85% of tumours greater than 2 cm have metastases). It is also related to tumour site. Metastases are rare in carcinoid of the appendix (3%), but common with those in the ileum (38%).

c) **True** Low-density lymphadenopathy is due to necrosis. Lymphadenopathy may be bulky and resemble lymphoma. Metastases to the liver are nearly always hypervascular and enhance early during the arterial phase. Metastases may also calcify. Other CT features include a stellate radiating pattern with beading of the mesenteric neurovascular bundle due to the desmoplastic reaction. There may be retraction and shortening of the mesentery with kinking and separation of the bowel loops.

d) **True** A second primary malignancy may be seen at another site in 36% of cases at autopsy.

e) **False** Multiple lesions may be seen in up to one third of cases.

40 a) **False** About 90% of bladder cancers are transitional cell tumours. Squamous cell carcinoma is associated with chronic infection (e.g. schistosomiasis) as well as calculi and leukoplakia. Risk factors for adenocarcinoma of the bladder include persistent urachus, cystitis glandularis and bladder exstrophy. Only 1%–2% of urachal abnormalities are complicated by squamous cell carcinoma. Only 1%–2% of urachal tumours are squamous cell neoplasms.

b) **True** MRI cannot distinguish invasion of the lamina propria from superficial muscle invasion, but can detect invasion into the deep muscle layer (T3 tumour).

c) **False** Transitional cell tumour may extend to the perivesical fat, seminal vesicles and prostate in males, but extension to the uterus and cervix is uncommon.

d) **False** The normal seminal vesicles are high signal on T2-weighted imaging. Low-signal changes may be seen with tumour extension, but also with atrophy, fibrosis and amyloid deposition. In the latter group, deposition tends to be bilateral and symmetrical. Tumour involvement is usually unilateral or asymmetrical. Alteration in morphology of the seminal vesicles may also indicate metastases.

e) **True** Early enhancement is related to tumour neovascularisation; typically, enhancement occurs within 2 minutes of intravenous gadolinium administration.

Chapter 4

Uroradiology

1 **Regarding the anatomy and development of the renal tract and adrenal gland, which of the following are true?**
   a) The adult kidney is formed directly from the mesonephros
   b) The mesonephric ducts in men lead to the development of the vas deferens
   c) There are usually three adrenal arteries and one adrenal vein bilaterally
   d) The bladder develops from the cloaca
   e) The posterior urethra in men is formed by the prostatic and bulbous segments

2 **Regarding ultrasound of the renal tract and adrenal glands, which of the following are true?**
   a) The normal renal cortex is more echogenic in neonates than in adults
   b) The neonatal adrenal glands are harder to visualise in neonates than in adults
   c) The junctional parenchymal defect is seen more commonly in the left kidney
   d) The renal resistive index is frequently normal in chronic obstruction
   e) The normal wall thickness of a well-distended bladder is less than 3 mm

3 **Concerning magnetic resonance imaging (MRI) of the kidneys and adrenal glands, which of the following are true?**
   a) Renal corticomedullary differentiation is more prominent on T2-weighted than T1-weighted imaging
   b) Gadolinium use is contraindicated in patients with impaired renal function
   c) Adrenal corticomedullary differentiation is not possible on MRI
   d) The adrenal glands demonstrate marked enhancement after intravenous gadolinium administration
   e) Following intravenous gadolinium administration, the urine may appear of low signal intensity on T2-weighted imaging

4 **Regarding congenital renal fusion anomalies, which of the following are true?**
   a) In a horseshoe kidney, the two kidneys are always joined at their inferior poles
   b) The renal pelvises point posteriorly in a horseshoe kidney
   c) There is a higher incidence of Wilms' tumour in a horseshoe kidney
   d) A pancake kidney results from fusion of both kidneys in the pelvis
   e) In crossed renal ectopia, renal fusion occurs in 85% of cases

5 **Which of the following are true of multicystic dysplastic kidneys?**
   a) Antenatal ultrasound reveals a paraspinal mass with multiple communicating cysts
   b) It is more common in infants of diabetic mothers
   c) Approximately 30% of contralateral kidneys are abnormal
   d) Up to 20% of cases have residual renal function in the affected kidney on scintigraphy
   e) Nephrectomy is usually required, as it cannot be differentiated from cystic Wilms' tumour

6 **Regarding multilocular cystic nephroma, which of the following are true?**
   a) It demonstrates autosomal dominant inheritance
   b) In females, it is more common after 4 years of age
   c) On computed tomography (CT), it typically has a poorly defined border with the rest of the kidney
   d) Enhancement or calcification of septae suggests a different diagnosis
   e) It is treated by nephrectomy

7   Which of the following conditions are associated with multiple renal cortical cysts?
   a) Caroli's disease
   b) Tuberous sclerosis
   c) Zellweger (cerebrohepatorenal) syndrome
   d) Turner's syndrome
   e) Dandy–Walker syndrome

8   Which of the following are true of adult polycystic kidney disease?
   a) It usually results from a defective gene on the short arm of chromosome 16
   b) The mean age of diagnosis is 20 years
   c) Females are more likely to develop associated hepatic cysts than males
   d) There is an association with mitral valve prolapse
   e) Antenatal ultrasound typically reveals enlarged kidneys with visible cysts

9   Regarding medullary sponge kidney, which of the following are true?
   a) The cystic areas in the medulla do not communicate with the collecting ducts
   b) The changes are unilateral in 25% of cases
   c) Medullary nephrocalcinosis is visible radiographically in 10% of cases
   d) It is a feature of Meckel–Gruber syndrome
   e) There is an association with Ehlers–Danlos syndrome

10 Concerning renal papillary necrosis, which of the following are true?
   a) Necrosis involves the overlying cortex in 10% of cases
   b) A single papilla is affected in approximately 15% of cases
   c) It is associated with a higher incidence of renal tract squamous cell carcinoma
   d) It may result from aspirin use
   e) Medullary sponge kidney is a cause

11 Cortical nephrocalcinosis is seen in which of the following?
   a) Ethylene glycol poisoning
   b) Chronic transplant rejection
   c) Chronic glomerulonephritis
   d) Oxalosis
   e) AIDS-related nephropathy

12 Medullary nephrocalcinosis occurs in which of the following conditions?
   a) Renal tubular acidosis
   b) Hyperparathyroidism
   c) Primary hyperoxaluria
   d) Secondary hyperoxaluria
   e) Lesch–Nyhan syndrome

13 Regarding renal calculi, which of the following are true?
   a) Renal calculi are more common in women than men
   b) More than 50% of staghorn calculi contain magnesium ammonium phosphate (struvite)
   c) Uric acid calculi are nonopaque
   d) Xanthine stones are not visible on CT
   e) Crohn's disease predisposes to the formation of oxalate stones

14 In xanthogranulomatous pyelonephritis, which of the following are true?
   a) About 75% of cases are associated with an underlying calculus
   b) About 90% of patients have diabetes mellitus
   c) The organism most commonly associated with the condition is *Escherichia coli*
   d) Imaging reveals a small kidney containing low attenuation parenchymal masses
   e) Optimal treatment is with antibiotics and percutaneous nephrostomy if there is associated obstruction

15 Regarding tuberculosis of the renal tract, which of the following are true?
   a) There is coexistent radiographic evidence of active pulmonary tuberculosis in 10% of cases
   b) Renal involvement is usually bilateral
   c) Involvement of the calyceal system is typically late in the disease process
   d) Vesico-ureteric reflux is uncommon because of ureteric stricture
   e) Bladder wall calcification is common

16 Which of the following are true of angiomyolipomas?
   a) Tumours are benign in 80% of cases
   b) Approximately 20%–40% of patients have tuberous sclerosis
   c) Calcification is present in less than 10% of cases
   d) On angiography, the lesions typically demonstrate arteriovenous shunting
   e) Nephrectomy is the treatment of choice, as underlying malignancy cannot be excluded

17 Which of the following are true of Wilms' tumour (nephroblastoma)?
   a) It is bilateral in one third of cases
   b) There is an association with sporadic aniridia
   c) Calcification is seen on CT in more than 50% of tumours
   d) Tumours are usually small at presentation
   e) Metastases to bone are common

18 Which of the following are true of renal cell carcinoma?
   a) von Hippel–Lindau syndrome is a risk factor
   b) Calcification and cystic change occur in the minority of cases
   c) About 75% of tumours less than 3 cm in size are hyperechoic on ultrasonography
   d) About 30% of tumours are hypovascular on angiography
   e) The lungs are the most common site for metastatic spread

19 Which of the following are true of renal neoplasms?
   a) Oncocytomas can be confidently differentiated from renal cell carcinoma on imaging
   b) Calcification is seen in 15% of oncocytomas
   c) Juxtaglomerular cell tumours (reninomas) are typically vascular tumours
   d) Renal involvement is more common in non-Hodgkin's lymphoma than Hodgkin's disease
   e) Metastases are the most common malignant tumour of the kidney

20 Regarding renal artery stenosis (RAS), which of the following are true?
   a) It is present in about 1%–2% of all patients with hypertension
   b) Atherosclerosis is the cause in more than 95% of cases in the developed world
   c) Fibromuscular dysplasia responds poorly to angioplasty
   d) A ratio of renal artery peak systolic velocity to aortic peak systolic velocity of more than 3.5 is suggestive of the diagnosis
   e) Haemodynamic significance is suggested by a trans-stenotic gradient of more than 40 mm Hg

21 Which of the following are true?
   a) Acute tubular necrosis following renal transplantation is more common in transplants with multiple renal arteries
   b) Perirenal fluid collections are seen in 10%–20% of transplants
   c) Transplant rejection typically leads to a fall in the resistive index
   d) In trauma, the absence of microscopic haematuria excludes a renal injury
   e) There is no parenchymal enhancement after a traumatic renal pedicle avulsion

22 Regarding congenital ureteric conditions, which of the following are true?
   a) Pelvi-ureteric junction obstruction is more common in females
   b) Pelvi-ureteric junction obstruction is more common on the left side
   c) In megaureter, there is dilatation of the distal ureter above a mechanical obstruction
   d) The abnormality in megaureter is bilateral in 80% of cases
   e) A retrocaval ureter occurs on the left side in 20% of cases

23 Which of the following are true regarding complete ureteric duplication?
   a) It is more common in males
   b) The orthotopic ureter drains the lower pole
   c) The upper moiety ureter is typically prone to vesico-ureteric reflux
   d) There are more calyces in the upper moiety collecting system
   e) In females, the ectopic ureter inserts below the external sphincter

24 Concerning ureterocoeles, which of the following are true?
   a) They can be indistinguishable from bladder diverticula during voiding
   b) A simple ureterocoele never occurs in an ectopic ureter
   c) A single simple ureterocoele can cause bladder outlet obstruction
   d) About 80% of ectopic ureterocoeles occur in duplicated systems
   e) In children, a pseudoureterocoele most commonly results from an impacted stone

25 Regarding vesico-ureteric reflux and reflux nephropathy, which of the following are true?
   a) Primary (congenital) vesico-ureteric reflux is seen in 30% of children with a single episode of urinary tract infection
   b) Secondary (acquired) vesico-ureteric reflux is seen in up to 50% of cases of cystitis
   c) A dilated and tortuous ureter in the presence of vesico-ureteric reflux is an indication for surgery
   d) Radionuclide cystography has a lower radiation dose than fluoroscopic cystography
   e) Renal scarring from reflux nephropathy is more common at the renal poles

26 Regarding pyeloureteritis cystica, which of the following are true?
   a) It is associated with recurrent ureteric calculi
   b) It is associated with diabetes mellitus
   c) It is characterised by multiple small epithelial outpouchings into the lamina propria
   d) It is usually bilateral
   e) The radiographic appearances resolve in the majority of cases after treatment

27 **Which of the following are true of retroperitoneal fibrosis?**
   a) The fibrotic plaque usually originates around the aortic bifurcation
   b) When the ureters are involved, there is typically only mild pyelocalyectasis
   c) On CT, the aorta is typically enveloped and anteriorly displaced by a fibrotic mass
   d) An increase in signal intensity on T2-weighted imaging indicates a good response to steroid treatment
   e) It is associated with primary sclerosing cholangitis

28 **In bladder exstrophy, which of the following are true?**
   a) There is frequently a bifid clitoris in affected females
   b) There is diastasis of the pubic symphysis
   c) In closed exstrophy, the mucosa of the bladder is continuous with the skin
   d) There is a frequent association with cryptorchidism
   e) There is an increased risk of bladder carcinoma

29 **In prune belly syndrome, which of the following are true?**
   a) The inheritance is autosomal recessive
   b) The condition is more common in females
   c) It is characterised by markedly distended and obstructed ureters
   d) There is an association with Hirschsprung's disease
   e) Death occurs within 1 year of birth in the majority of cases

30 **Concerning bladder neoplasia, which of the following are true?**
   a) Analgesic abuse is a risk factor for bladder transitional cell carcinoma
   b) Bladder exstrophy is a risk factor for squamous cell carcinoma
   c) Urachal carcinoma calcifies in 70% of cases
   d) Leiomyoma is the most common type of benign bladder tumour
   e) Bladder involvement is more common in non-Hodgkin's than Hodgkin's disease

31 **Regarding trauma to the bladder, which of the following are true?**
   a) Approximately 10% of patients with a pelvic fracture have associated bladder injury
   b) Bladder contusion is the most common form of traumatic bladder injury
   c) About 50% of bladder ruptures are intraperitoneal
   d) Extraperitoneal ruptures are most common around the base of the bladder
   e) About 10% of bladder ruptures are only evident on postvoiding cystography films

32 **Regarding infection of the urinary tract, which of the following are true?**
   a) *Schistosoma mansoni* causes bladder wall calcification
   b) Malakoplakia most commonly involves the bladder
   c) Leukoplakia most commonly involves the bladder
   d) About 20%–40% of cases of emphysematous pyelonephritis result from ureteral obstruction
   e) Patients with AIDS nephropathy have an increased risk of developing renal cell carcinoma

33 Regarding the urethra, which of the following are true?
a) The bladder neck is typically dilated on cystography in patients with posterior urethral valves
b) A short well-defined stricture favours a noninfective aetiology
c) Trauma to the anterior urethra is more common than to the posterior urethra
d) Transitional cell carcinoma is the most common primary malignant tumour
e) Acquired urethral diverticula are more common in females

34 Which of the following are true of prostate cancer?
a) Benign prostatic hypertrophy (BPH) predisposes to prostate cancer
b) Serum prostate specific antigen (PSA) levels can be elevated by BPH
c) Low signal on T2-weighted imaging within the seminal vesicle is diagnostic of seminal vesical invasion
d) About 40% of hypoechoic peripheral zone lesions on transrectal ultrasound are malignant
e) Pelvic side wall lymph nodes more than 8 mm in the short axis are abnormal

35 Regarding endorectal MRI of the prostate, which of the following are true?
a) Routine use of contrast enhancement is essential in the staging of prostate cancer
b) The endorectal surface coil does not allow assessment of all pelvic nodes
c) MRI spectroscopy has no current role in the diagnosis of prostate carcinoma
d) On T2-weighted imaging, the peripheral zone appears hyperintense
e) Capsular bulging strongly suggests extracapsular tumour spread

36 Regarding testicular ultrasound, which of the following are true?
a) The normal epididymis is slightly hypoechoic to the normal testis
b) There is an association between testicular microlithiasis and Klinefelter's syndrome
c) Testicular cysts are seen in up to 10% of testicular ultrasound studies
d) The epididymis is typically enlarged, hypervascular and hyperechoic when inflamed
e) Absent testicular blood flow on colour Doppler imaging is pathognomonic of testicular torsion

37 Regarding the malpositioned testis, which of the following are true?
a) About 10% of testes are maldescended in neonates delivered at term
b) Cryptorchidism is associated with Noonan's syndrome
c) Cryptorchidism is bilateral in 10% of cases
d) There is an increased risk of testicular torsion in cryptorchidism
e) Teratoma is the most common tumour in undescended testes

38 Which of the following are true of testicular neoplasms?
a) A contralateral tumour develops in 8% of cases
b) Germ cell tumours account for 75% of all testicular neoplasms
c) Teratoma is the most common germ cell tumour
d) Choriocarcinoma classically metastasises late
e) Metastases to the testes are more common than germ cell tumours in patients aged more than 55 years

39 Regarding phaeochromocytoma, which of the following are true?

a) The incidence of malignancy is lower in extra-adrenal compared to adrenal phaeochromocytoma
b) Extra-adrenal tumours occur most commonly at the aortic bifurcation
c) There is an association with parathyroid adenoma
d) MIBG scintigraphy has a 10% false negative rate for tumour detection
e) They are high signal on T2-weighted imaging and enhance avidly after gadolinium administration

40 Regarding adrenal cortical carcinoma, which of the following are true?

a) This is the most common primary malignant adrenal tumour
b) There is an association with hemihypertrophy
c) Excess hormone production is present in at least 50% of patients
d) They are bilateral in 30% of cases
e) These tumours are usually radiosensitive

Answers

1 a) **False** The adult kidney is formed from the metanephros (metanephric blastema) under the influence of the ureteral bud, which comes off the caudal end of the mesonephric duct.

b) **True** In men, these ducts form the vas deferens, seminal vesicles and ejaculatory ducts, whereas in women they undergo complete involution.

c) **True** Normal arterial supply is via the superior (branch of the inferior phrenic artery), middle (from aorta) and inferior (from renal artery) adrenal arteries. Each gland is drained by a single vein, which enters the inferior vena cava (IVC) on the right and the renal vein on the left.

d) **True** The cloaca is divided by the urorectal septum into an anterior urogenital sinus and a posterior rectum (failure of this process leads to bladder agenesis). The urogenital sinus develops into the bladder and urethra (and prostate).

e) **False** In men, the urethra is divided into posterior (made up of prostatic and membranous) and anterior (made up of bulbous and penile) segments. The female urethra is divided into intrapelvic, membranous and perineal parts.

2 a) **True** Glomeruli occupy a greater proportion of the cortex in the neonate, appearing more echogenic than the adjacent liver and spleen. The converse is true in adults.

b) **False** Relative to renal size the adrenal glands are much larger in neonates. The right is normally easier to visualise than the left.

c) **False** The junctional parenchymal defect is an echogenic notch in the renal cortical contour that may extend to the sinus and results from incomplete fusion of the two sub-kidneys. It is more commonly seen in children, in the right kidney and at the junction of the middle and upper thirds, and should not be mistaken for a scar.

d) **True** The resistive index can be elevated in obstruction (greater than 0.75, and more than 0.08 higher than the nonobstructed side). However, the resistive index can be elevated by nonobstructive renal disease as well as being normal in chronic obstruction.

e) **True** The normal wall thickness of a well-distended bladder is usually less or equal to 5 mm in a nondistended bladder. Wall thickening is seen with: tumours, infection and inflammation (cystitis), muscular hypertrophy (neurogenic bladder and outlet obstruction) and underdistended bladders.

3 a) **False** The converse is true. On T1-weighted imaging, there is distinct corticomedullary differentiation with the cortex having a medium signal intensity (similar to liver) and the medulla having lower signal intensity. On moderate T2-weighted imaging, corticomedullary differentiation is not usually seen and both cortex and medulla are hyperintense. On heavily T2-weighted images, the medulla is slightly more intense than the cortex.

b) **False** Although 95% is excreted via the kidneys (5% hepatobiliary), intravenous gadolinium can be safely used in renal impairment, although the excretion is prolonged (normal $t_{1/2}$ = 90 minutes).

c) **True** Adrenal corticomedullary differentiation is also not possible on CT. However, the adrenal medulla appears as a linear echogenic structure on ultrasonography in neonates.

d) **False** There is only slight enhancement of the adrenal glands after intravenous gadolinium administration.

e) **True** This reflects the very high concentrations of excreted gadolinium in urine, which can lead to a fall in signal intensity (most often seen in renal pelvis and bladder).

4 a) **False** The two kidneys are joined (upper poles in 10% and lower poles in 90%) by a parenchymal or fibrous band, which lies at L4/5 between the aorta and inferior mesenteric artery. It is the most common renal fusion anomaly (1–4 per 1000 births) and is more common in males. There is an association with pelvi-ureteric obstruction, ureteral duplication and malformations of the cardiovascular system, musculoskeletal system and anorectal region.

b) **False** The renal pelvises point anteriorly. The ureters descend in front of the isthmus.

c) **True** There is also an increased risk of trauma, calculi, obstruction and infection in a horseshoe kidney.

d) **True** Fusion is usually near the aortic bifurcation. The associations include: cryptorchidism, vaginal or sacral agenesis, caudal regression and tetralogy of Fallot.

e) **True** In crossed renal ectopia the kidney is located on the opposite side of midline to its ureteral orifice. Four types have been described: crossed renal ectopia with fusion, without fusion, solitary crossed renal ectopia (only one kidney, which lies contralateral to its ureteral orifice) and bilateral crossed renal ectopia (both kidneys are crossed). The left kidney is more likely to cross than the right. The crossed kidney is inferior to the normal kidney. Associations include megaureter, hypospadias and multicystic dysplastic kidney.

5 a) **False** The cysts are typically noncommunicating and of variable size, allowing differentiation from hydronephrosis. Multicystic dysplastic kidney is the second most common cause of neonatal abdominal mass after hydronephrosis. It results from complete ureteral obstruction (at 8–10 weeks' gestational age), which inhibits nephron maturation and the collecting tubules enlarge into cysts.

   b) **True** The incidence is 1:4000 for unilateral multicystic dysplastic kidney and 1:10000 when bilateral. It is unilateral in 80% of cases. It is also associated with Turner's syndrome.

   c) **True** The most common contralateral renal abnormalities are pelvi-ureteric junction obstruction, horseshoe kidney or vesico-ureteric reflux. Ipsilateral anomalies include vesico-ureteric reflux (in 25% of cases) and an ectopic ureter.

   d) **True** Residual renal function is seen best on delayed scans.

   e) **False** Serial ultrasound scans of multicystic dysplastic kidney usually show renal involution. There is a small risk of renin-dependent hypertension. Malignant change is rare (less than 0.5%). Nephrectomy is only required if it fails to involute, or if there is uncontrolled hypertension.

6 a) **False** It is a rare nonhereditary benign neoplasm, which is usually large and contains multiple noncommunicating cysts with prominent septae. No association with congenital anomalies in other organ systems has been established.

   b) **True** It has a biphasic age and sex distribution – female patients with multilocular cystic nephroma typically present with symptoms between 4 and 20 years of age or after 40 years of age. Conversely, 90% of tumours in males occur in the first 2 years of life. Consequently, among children presenting before 4 years of age, over 70% are male whereas nearly 90% of patients presenting after 4 years of age are female.

   c) **False** The lesion is unifocal and encapsulated, with a well-defined border to the adjacent normal kidney. Hence, it can be differentiated from multicystic dysplastic kidney, which normally involves the whole kidney and, when focal, is ill defined.

   d) **False** The septae often calcify and may enhance.

   e) **True** It is surgically removed because distinction from cystic Wilms' tumour is not possible by imaging. Local recurrence or coexistent Wilms' tumour is very rare.

7 **All true** Cortical cysts are very common (50% incidence in those aged over 50 years) and arise from obstructed tubules or ducts. They do not communicate with the collecting system (unlike pyelogenic cysts) and are most commonly asymptomatic, but can cause haematuria, infection, pain and even hypertension. Cortical cysts should be differentiated from medullary cystic disease, which is a spectrum of diseases with various inheritance patterns (autosomal recessive and autosomal dominant), which have juvenile and adult onsets and an association with retinitis pigmentosa. They frequently lead to renal failure and are characterised by medullary cysts (small and often not resolved on imaging) and a thin cortex free of cysts. Syndromes associated with multiple renal cortical cysts include Meckel–Gruber, Jeune's, trisomy 13, von Hippel–Lindau, Conradi's disease (chondrodystrophia congenital punctata) and uraemic cystic disease (seen in 90% of patients on dialysis for more than 5 years).

8 a) **True**   Inheritance is usually autosomal dominant, but spontaneous mutations occur in 10% of cases. In 85%–95% of cases, patients have a genetic abnormality at 16p13.3 and this gene has been named PKD1. A second gene named PKD2 lies at 4q21–23; patients with this gene tend to have a milder form of disease.

    b) **False**   There is great variability in onset of cystic change. Mean age at diagnosis is 45 years for PKD1 and 69 years for PKD2.

    c) **True**   Liver cysts develop in 25%–75% of patients. Females are more commonly and severely affected than males. The cysts may be sensitive to sustained levels of sex hormones because cyst size is related to parity of the patient.

    d) **True**   Cysts may also be detected in other organs such as the pancreas (10% of cases) and spleen (less than 5% of cases). Cysts may rarely occur within the lungs, thyroid, ovaries, uterus and scrotum. Saccular berry aneurysms of cerebral arteries are present in up to 20% of cases.

    e) **False**   Visualisation of the cysts at this stage is unusual. The kidneys appear enlarged and diffusely echogenic with a poorly demarcated renal contour.

9 a) **False**   This is a relatively common sporadic condition affecting mainly young-to-middle-aged adults. There is dysplastic cystic dilatation of papillary and medullary portions of the collecting ducts.

    b) **True**   The process may involve one or both kidneys or may be confined to a single papilla. It is often asymptomatic, but it may be complicated by stones, haematuria or infection. Less than 10% of cases result in renal impairment.

    c) **False**   Medullary nephrocalcinosis is visible radiographically in 40%–80% of cases. A striated nephrogram on excretory urogram is typical.

    d) **False**   This autosomal recessive syndrome is characterised by bilateral multicystic dysplastic kidneys, occipital encephalocoele and polydactyly.

    e) **True**   Other associations include hemihypertrophy, parathyroid adenoma, Caroli's disease, congenital pyloric stenosis and other renal lesions.

10 a) **False**   The cortex is never involved. Renal papillary necrosis results from an ischaemic coagulative necrosis of the pyramids and medullary papilla secondary to interstitial nephritis or intrinsic vascular obstruction.

    b) **True**   Renal papillary necrosis can be localised/diffuse and unilateral/bilateral. Multiple papillae are affected in 85% of cases. Bilateral disease usually reflects a systemic illness.

    c) **True**   In addition, there is an eight-fold increase of transitional cell carcinoma in analgesic abusers.

    d) **True**   Analgesics are one of the most common causes of renal papillary necrosis. Other causes include: diabetes mellitus, sickle cell disease, pyelonephritis, obstructive uropathy, tuberculosis, trauma, alcohol and renal vein thrombosis.

    e) **False**   Medullary sponge kidney is a condition characterised by dysplastic dilatation of the collecting tubules. It causes renal papillary calculi but not necrosis.

11 All true Cortical nephrocalcinosis (5% of cases) is much less common than medullary nephrocalcinosis (95% of cases). It is characterised by peripheral (occasionally tramline) calcification, which spares the medullary pyramids. The columns of Bertin may be involved. Ultrasonography shows a hyperechoic cortex. Other causes include acute cortical necrosis (secondary to pregnancy, shock, infections and toxins, such as methoxyfluorane and ethylene glycol), Alport's syndrome and chronic hypercalcaemia.

12 All true This form of nephrocalcinosis results from a diffuse process and is characterised by calcification of the distal convoluted tubules and the loops of Henle. Imaging reveals stippled pyramidal calcification and a hyperechoic medulla. Other causes include medullary sponge kidney (which along with renal tubular acidosis and hyperparathyroidism accounts for 70% of all causes), renal papillary necrosis, any cause of hypercalcaemia/hypercalciuria (such as milk–alkali syndrome, sarcoidosis, frusemide therapy, vitamin E or calcium supplements and Bartter's syndrome) and any cause of hyperuricosuria (such as gouty kidney or Lesch–Nyhan syndrome).

13 a) False The reverse is true. Calculi are four times more common in men. Struvite stones are the exception to this rule, as they are twice as common in women. About 12% of the population develop stones by age 70 years and 2%–3% of the population experience an attack of renal colic. Stones recur in 50% of untreated patients within 10 years. About 80% of all stones contain calcium oxalate or calcium phosphate.

   b) True Struvite calculi account for 70% of staghorn calculi (the remainder are cystine or uric acid stones) and are commonly the result of urea-splitting organisms such as *Proteus*. Struvite is usually mixed with calcium phosphate to create 'triple phosphate' calculi.

   c) True Other nonopaque stones include xanthine and the rare mucoprotein matrix calculi, which occur in poorly functioning, infected urinary tracts. Cystine calculi are slightly opaque.

   d) False CT detects most calculi regardless of composition, although matrix stones are poorly visualised. Contiguous unenhanced images are required. A stone in the ureter often has a rim of surrounding soft tissue from mucosal oedema (ureteric rim sign), which helps to differentiate it from phlebolith. However, stones resulting from indinavir treatment (in HIV seropositive patients) are frequently lucent even on CT.

   e) True The formation of oxalate stones is secondary to excess oxalate absorption from the bowel, which also occurs in ulcerative colitis and following a small bowel bypass or resection. These patients are also at an increased risk of uric acid stones.

14 a) **True** In 75% of cases, there is an underlying stone, which causes obstruction and chronic inflammation/infection with subsequent parenchymal destruction and deposition of lipid-laden macrophages. The remaining cases result from a pelvi-ureteric obstruction or a ureteric tumour. The kidney is diffusely involved in 90% of cases.

b) **False** Approximately 10% of patients have diabetes mellitus.

c) **False** *Proteus* is the most commonly associated organism. *E. coli, Klebsiella, Pseudomonas* and *Enterobacter* are also frequently cultured. Multiorganism urinary tract infection is common.

d) **False** The kidney is irregularly enlarged with parenchymal replacement by xanthomatous masses (CT: –10 to 30 HU) that may extend into the perinephric space.

e) **False** Optimal treatment involves nephrectomy.

15 a) **True** Only 5%–15% of cases have active cavitary tuberculosis. The renal tract is the second most common site of tuberculous involvement after the lungs. Renal disease typically results from haematogenous spread from the lung, bone or gastrointestinal tract. Frequency, sterile pyuria and haematuria are common presenting symptoms.

b) **False** Involvement is unilateral in 70% of cases. Infection commences within the renal parenchyma, which ulcerates into the collecting system and may descend down the renal tract. Imaging findings include calcification (autonephrectomy in advanced cases), cavity formation, scarring, papillary necrosis and tuberculomas (20% of cases).

c) **False** Involvement of the calyceal system is early with mucosal irregularity, infundibular stenoses and amputated calyces. Renal calculi are present in 10% of cases.

d) **False** Vesico-ureteric reflux is common through the fixed patulous ureteric orifice.

e) **False** Calcification of the bladder wall can occur but is rare. Wall thickening and ulceration with a 'shrunken' bladder are more usual. Calcification may also be observed within the seminal vesicles and epididymis. Infection is not associated with an increased risk of renal cell carcinoma.

16 a) **False** Tumours are always benign. Angiomyolipomas are hamartomas composed of varying amounts of fat, smooth muscle and thick-walled blood vessels. The blood vessels lack a complete elastic layer and this predisposes to bleeding and aneurysm formation. Lesions more than 4 cm in size bleed spontaneously in 50%–60% of cases.

b) **True** Conversely, angiomyolipomas occur in 80% of patients with tuberous sclerosis (commonly multiple).

c) **True** Calcification is rare and probably reflects previous haemorrhage. A renal lesion containing fat is very suggestive of an angiomyolipoma, although there are a few case reports of fat within renal cell carcinomas and oncocytomas.

d) **False** Arteriovenous shunting is rarely seen and is more typical of renal cell carcinoma. About 95% of cases are hypervascular with enlarged and tortuous vessels.

e) **False** Small lesions (less than 4 cm) are followed-up annually, whilst larger lesions can be treated with either a partial nephrectomy or selective embolisation.

17 a) **False** Wilms' tumour is the most common intra-abdominal malignancy in children. It is the third most common paediatric malignancy after brain tumours and leukaemia. The mean age of presentation is about 3 years old. It is bilateral in 5%–10% of cases. The disease may be multifocal in 10% of cases. About 50% of cases occur in children under the age of 2 years and 75% occur under the age of 5 years. Nephroblastomatosis is a precursor.

b) **True** About 15% of patients with Wilms' tumour have an associated syndrome or clinical problem. Of patients with Beckwith–Wiedemann syndrome, 10%–20% develop Wilms' tumour. Up to 33% of patients with sporadic aniridia develop Wilms' tumour. There are also strong associations with Drash syndrome, pseudohermaphroditism, glomerulonephritis, and nephrotic syndrome and hemihypertrophy. There have been reports of increased incidence with neurofibromatosis (NF), Bloom's syndrome, horseshoe kidneys, hypospadias and cryptorchidism. Patients with Beckwith–Wiedemann syndrome, sporadic aniridia and hemihypertrophy tend to present younger and have bilateral disease.

c) **False** Calcification is seen in 15% of cases (5% on plain films) on CT. This helps to differentiate Wilms' tumours from neuroblastomas (in which calcification is seen in 85%–95% of cases). Other features in favour of a Wilms' tumour include: intrinsic renal mass effect (instead of displacement), older age of onset (neuroblastoma normally occurs under 2 years), absence of vascular involvement (neuroblastomas frequently encase midline vessels) and unilaterality (neuroblastomas are bilateral in more than 50% of cases).

d) **False** About 90% of cases in children present with a palpable abdominal mass, which is often asymptomatic. Most tumours are large (more than 12 cm) at presentation. Haematuria is common (20% of cases). The incidence of hypertension varies from 15% to 90%, which may be due to renin production or vascular compression.

e) **False** Bone metastases are rare. Common secondary sites are the lung and liver.

18 a) **True** Other risk factors include tobacco, long-term phenacetin use, chronic haemodialysis (more than 3 years) and a family history.

b) **True** Calcification occurs in 5%–20% of tumours and is usually central and amorphous, but may be peripheral or curvilinear in cystic renal cell carcinoma. Cystic change occurs in 2%–15% of cases.

c) **True** Tumours larger than 3 cm in size tend to be isoechoic or hypoechoic.

d) **False** Only 5% of tumours are hypovascular on angiography. Tumours cause neovascularity, which on angiography may lead to contrast puddling, arteriovenous shunting, small aneurysms and parasitisation of other vessels. Tumour growth into the renal vein (20%–35%) or IVC (5%–10%) may be seen.

e) **True** About 55% of all metastatic deposits occur in the lungs. Other sites include: the liver (35%), bone (30%; classically lytic and expansile), adrenals (20%), contralateral kidney (10%) and other organs (less than 5%).

19 a) False These tumours have a peak incidence in the seventh decade. They arise from the epithelial cells (oncocytes) of the proximal convoluted tubule (2%–10% of all renal tumours). They are benign, but they may have to be removed, as confident differentiation from renal cell carcinoma may not be possible preoperatively. The majority of patients are asymptomatic.

b) False Calcification is rare. Classical imaging findings include a well-defined low-density mass with pseudocapsule. On ultrasonography, more than 50% of cases are hypoechoic. A central scar is visible in 30% of cases. On angiography, 80% of cases demonstrate a spoke wheel configuration, but no arteriovenous shunting.

c) False These rare tumours are typically small (less than 3 cm), appearing hypovascular or avascular on angiography and enhancing less well than normal kidney on CT. They may appear echogenic on ultrasonography.

d) True There are three patterns of lymphomatous involvement: primary renal lymphoma (rare as the kidneys lack lymphatic tissue), haematogenous dissemination (common) and direct spread from the retroperitoneum (common). On imaging, multiple hypoechoic or hypodense nodules are the most common finding. The disease may also appear as a single mass or diffuse infiltration.

e) True Metastases are 2–3 times as frequent as primary tumours in the kidney at autopsy. Primary sites include lung, breast, colon, the opposite kidney and melanoma.

20 a) True RAS is also present in 25% of patients with difficult-to-control hypertension.

b) False Atherosclerosis accounts for about 70%–90% of cases, with the remaining resulting from fibromuscular dysplasia (10%–30%), NF, arteritis (polyarteritis nodosa, Takayasu's arteritis, Buerger's disease, congenital rubella), radiotherapy, aortic dissection/aneurysm, arteriovenous fistula, phaeochromocytoma and retroperitoneal fibrosis.

c) False Fibromuscular dysplasia responds well to angioplasty and tends to affect the mid and distal thirds of the renal artery (compared with atherosclerosis, which affects the proximal 2 cm of renal artery and responds less well to angioplasty). Fibromuscular dysplasia is the most common cause of renal artery stenosis in children.

d) True Other suggestive signs include a renal artery peak systolic velocity of more than 180 cm/second, poststenotic spectral broadening, absent end-diastolic blood flow and a tardus-parvus pattern in the distal artery. The role of ultrasonography in screening is controversial because of technical difficulties (inadvertent sampling of adjacent collateral vessels), incomplete examination(s) (up to 50% of cases) or the presence of multiple renal arteries (25% of cases).

e) True Other signs indicating that a stenosis is haemodynamically significant include: a more than 70% stenosis, poststenotic dilatation, the presence of collateral vessels, a small kidney and finally a ratio of renin levels, on venous sampling, between the affected and unaffected renal veins of more than 1.5 (not valid in the presence of bilateral stenoses).

21 a) **True** Acute tubular necrosis is also more common in cadaveric transplants (due to donor hypotension, which is seen less with living related donors) and transplants with prolonged organ storage. Scintigraphic flow may be normal, but there is diminished excretion. Ultrasonography demonstrates smooth enlarged kidneys, elevated resistive index (more than 0.7) and echogenic pyramids. Acute tubular necrosis is most commonly seen in the first 24 hours following transplant and rarely occurs after 1 month (compared with cyclosporin toxicity which looks similar to acute tubular necrosis on imaging, but rarely occurs in the first month).

b) **False** Perirenal fluid collections are present in up to 50% of transplants. These may be lymphocoeles (10%–20% of cases; usually inferomedial to the kidney, large with thick septa in 50%–80% of cases and internal echoes), urinoma (rarely septated and smaller than lymphocoeles), abscess (fever and complex) or haematoma (hyperechoic on ultrasonography).

c) **False** This fall in the RI may result initially from an autoregulatory mechanism. With time, the typical finding of an elevated resistive index develops. Although values between 0.7 and 0.9 are nonspecific and can also be seen in acute tubular necrosis, values above 0.9 have a more than 95% positive predictive value for rejection.

d) **False** With renal pedicle avulsion, the nonperfused kidney may not produce urine. Furthermore, ureteric avulsion may prevent blood-stained urine reaching the bladder.

e) **False** There is enhancement of the renal periphery through intact capsular vessels (rim sign). Pedicle avulsion is seen in 5% of cases of renal trauma and is treated surgically. Other forms of renal trauma include subcapsular haematoma, renal contusion, superficial renal laceration (all treated conservatively) and complete laceration that communicates with the calyceal system (management is controversial; 15%–50% will require surgery).

22 a) **False** It is five times more common in males than females, resulting from either a functional obstruction (80% of cases), secondary to a defect in the circular muscle of the renal pelvis, or from extrinsic compression (20% of cases).

b) **True** It may also be bilateral in 10%–40% of cases. The contralateral kidney is absent in 10% of cases and dysplastic in 25%. It is the most common cause of neonatal hydronephrosis.

c) **False** There is functional obstruction of the distal ureter secondary to abnormal muscular development (achalasia of ureter). This results in an aperistaltic localised dilatation of the pelvic ureter with smooth tapered narrowing of the intravesical ureter. It is the second most common cause of neonatal hydronephrosis.

d) **False** The condition is more frequent in males. It is bilateral in 20%–40% of cases, but is more common on the left side. Contralateral renal abnormalities such as pelvi-ureteric obstruction, reflux, ureterocoele, ureteric duplication, renal ectopia and renal agenesis may occur.

e) **False** Retrocaval ureter is a right-sided condition and is three times more common in males. The ureter passes behind the IVC and exits between the aorta and IVC. It results from persistence of the right subcardinal vein with medial looping of the right ureter at L3. Obstruction may occur.

23 a) **False** Complete ureteric duplication is twice as common in females and is bilateral in 15%–40% of cases. Complete duplication results from a second ureteral bud arising from the mesonephric duct. Incomplete duplication results from branching of a single ureteral bud before it reaches the developing kidney.

b) **True** In complete ureteric duplication, the lower pole ureter enters the bladder normally, while the upper pole ureter has an ectopic insertion (Weigert–Meyer rule).

c) **False** The upper moiety ureter is prone to obstruction and ureterocoele formation while the lower moiety ureter is prone to reflux.

d) **False** The upper collecting system usually consists of only one major calyx.

e) **True** This may result in urinary incontinence, as the ureter may insert into the distal urethra, vagina and uterus. In males, the ureteric insertion is suprasphincteric.

24 a) **True** A ureterocoele is a cystic ectatic subepithelial segment of distal ureter that prolapses into the bladder; on urography, it is seen as a typical smooth thin 'cobra head' deformity. On voiding, a ureterocoele may evert and resemble a diverticulum.

b) **True** By definition, simple (orthotopic) ureterocoeles occur in normally located ureters. They are more common in females, are usually found in single systems and are frequently unilateral (80% of cases), asymptomatic and incidental findings.

c) **True** A simple ureterocoele may rarely prolapse into the bladder neck or urethra causing obstruction. It can also result in ureteric dilatation or stone formation.

d) **True** Only 20% of ectopic ureteroceles occur in single systems. They are bilateral in 10% of cases. When large, they can cause obstruction of the bladder outlet or the contralateral ureter.

e) **True** A pseudoureterocoele is an obstructed, but otherwise normal, intramural ureter that mimics a ureterocoele. It can be differentiated from a ureterocoele on urography. The halo is thick and irregular and the lesions are acquired. The causes include transitional cell carcinoma (the most common cause in adults), invasion by cervical cancer, and oedema resulting from stone, radiation or instrumentation.

25 a) **True** Hence the need for a low index of suspicion. Primary reflux results from immaturity of the vesico-ureteric junction with an abnormally short submucosal ureteral tunnel through the bladder wall.

b) **True** Secondary (acquired) reflux can also result from ureteric duplication with a ureterocoele, paraureteric (Hutch) diverticulum, posterior urethral valves, neurogenic bladder and absent abdominal musculature (prune belly syndrome).

c) **True** Clubbed and dilated calyces (Grade IV reflux) or a dilated tortuous ureter (Grade V reflux) are indications for surgery. Reflux into just the distal ureter (Grade I) or a collecting system that is of normal calibre (Grade II) or only mildly dilated (Grade III) is likely to resolve spontaneously as the vesico-ureteric junction matures. Primary reflux improves spontaneously in 80% of cases.

d) **True** Two varieties of radionuclide cystography may be performed: indirect with intravenous injection of technetium-99m diethylenetriaminepentaacetic acid (^{99m}Tc DTPA) and direct with bladder instillation of ^{99m}Tc pertechnetate.

e) **True** Scarring results from the intrarenal reflux of infected urine from the collecting system into the renal parenchyma. Compound papillae (common at the renal poles) have collecting ducts with prominent orificia and hence are more susceptible to scarring.

26 a) **True**   Pyeloureteritis cystica is a result of chronic urinary tract infection or stone disease. It is more common in females.

b) **True**   Patients with diabetes mellitus are predisposed to pyeloureteritis cystica.

c) **False**   This describes ureteral pseudodiverticulosis. In pyeloureteritis cystica, small fluid-filled mural cysts develop and project into the lumen of the pelvis and ureter. The cysts are usually 1–5 mm in diameter, but may reach up to 2 cm.

d) **False**   Pyeloureteritis cystica is usually unilateral. The condition is most common in the bladder, followed by the proximal third of the ureter and the pelvi-ureteric junction.

e) **False**   The condition may resolve with antibiotic treatment, but frequently persists unchanged for years. It is associated with an increased incidence of transitional cell carcinoma.

27 a) **True**   The fibrotic plaque begins around the aortic bifurcation and extends up to the renal hilum with effects on the ureters, lymphatics and great vessels. It rarely extends below the pelvic brim. The incidence in males is twice that of females and the condition generally occurs between the ages of 30 and 60 years.

b) **True**   Evidence shows that obstruction relates to interference with ureteric peristalsis rather than mechanical effects. Medial deviation of the ureter on urography is typical.

c) **False**   The aorta is engulfed by a fibrotic mass, but not displaced. Displacement is more typical of retroperitoneal malignancies, such as lymphoma.

d) **False**   A decrease in tissue oedema after steroid treatment is reflected by a reduction in signal intensity on T2-weighted MRI.

e) **True**   Primary disease (two thirds of cases) is thought to result from an autoimmune vasculitis due to antibodies to ceroid, a by-product of aortic plaque. In approximately 10% of cases, it is associated with fibrosis elsewhere, including the mediastinum, thyroid, biliary tree and orbit. Secondary retroperitoneal fibrosis can result from drugs (e.g. methysergide, methyldopa and ergotamine), malignancy induced desmoplasia (e.g. lymphoma, carcinoid and metastases), haematoma and polyarteritis nodosa.

28 a) **True**   Bladder exstrophy results from incomplete retraction of the cloacal membrane and is characterised by a defect in the lower abdominal wall and pubic region with the urinary bladder exposed and open anteriorly. In males, the defect in the dorsal aspect of the urethra causes epispadias.

b) **True**   The width of the diastasis correlates with the degree of the exstrophy. Other congenital causes of a widened symphysis include cleidocranial dysostosis, cloacal exstrophy, prune belly syndrome and osteogenesis imperfecta.

c) **False**   In closed exstrophy (pseudoexstrophy), there is persistence of the cloacal membrane. The anterior bladder wall lies subcutaneously and is covered by a thin epithelial membrane.

d) **True**   Other associated conditions include a low-lying umbilicus, omphalocele, inguinal hernia, clubfoot, imperforate anus and cardiac anomalies.

e) **True**   Bladder carcinoma develops in 4% of patients.

29 a) **False** Prune belly syndrome is a sporadic nonhereditary condition.

  b) **False** It occurs almost exclusively in males.

  c) **False** It is characterised by the triad of absent or hypoplastic abdominal wall musculature (causes prune belly appearance), nonobstructed markedly distended redundant ureters and cryptorchidism (bladder distension interferes with testicular descent). There is a spectrum of severity.

  d) **True** Other associations include: urethral atresia, dysplastic kidneys, vesico-ureteric reflux, oligohydramnios and pulmonary hypoplasia, patent urachus, congenital heart disease, congenital cystoadenomatoid malformation of the lung and multiple skeletal abnormalities.

  e) **False** In 20% of cases, death occurs in the first month of life. In another 30%, death occurs within 2 years of birth. Mild cases survive into adulthood.

30 a) **True** Other risk factors include smoking, aniline dyes, aromatic amines, azo dyes in rubber manufacturing, pelvic radiation and cyclophosphamide therapy. Transitional cell carcinoma accounts for 90% of all bladder tumours.

  b) **False** Bladder exstrophy is a risk factor for bladder adenocarcinoma, which accounts for only 2% of bladder tumours, along with cystitis glandularis and a urachal remnant. Risk factors for squamous cell carcinoma (5% of tumours) include: calculi, chronic infection or instrumentation, bladder diverticula, leukoplakia and schistosomiasis.

  c) **True** Urachal carcinoma calcifies in 70% of cases, unlike bladder transitional cell carcinoma, which calcifies in less than 10% of cases. Urachal carcinoma is a rare tumour, which occurs in adolescence (70% occur before age 20 years) and arises from the urachal remnant in the midline.

  d) **True** Leiomyoma lesions are usually submucosal and occur around the trigone.

  e) **True** Bladder involvement is usually seen in disseminated disease. Primary bladder lymphoma is rare (1% of bladder tumours) and usually occurs around the base or trigone.

31 a) **True** There are four main types of bladder injury: bladder contusion, interstitial bladder rupture (rare, incomplete serosal perforation with intact mucosa), intraperitoneal rupture and extraperitoneal rupture. Combinations may occur.

  b) **True** Bladder contusion represents a nonperforating tear of the bladder mucosa resulting in an intramural haematoma. Cystography can be normal, but may show lack of normal bladder distensibility or a crescent-shaped filling defect.

  c) **False** Only 20% of bladder ruptures are intraperitoneal and such cases generally result from either a blunt trauma to a distended bladder or a penetrating injury, such as cystoscopy or a stab wound. It occurs at the dome of the bladder. Cystography reveals contrast around bowel loops and in paracolic gutters.

  d) **True** Such ruptures are due to bony spicula from the pelvic fracture or an avulsion tear at the insertion of the puboprostatic ligaments. They account for up to 80% of ruptures. Cystography reveals contrast leakage around the bladder base, which sometimes extends into the thigh or abdominal wall. The bladder appears pear-shaped on plain film.

  e) **True** Cystography may miss ruptures sealed by haematoma or mesentery.

32 a) **False** *S. mansoni,* along with *S. japonicum,* affects the gastrointestinal tract and causes portal hypertension. *S. haematobium* involves the urinary tract and causes bladder wall calcification, which may extend up the ureters. Other causes of bladder wall calcification include tuberculosis, cyclophosphamide-induced cystitis, interstitial cystitis, radiotherapy and bladder neoplasm.

b) **True** However, malakoplakia can affect any part of the urinary tract from the kidney to the testes and/or prostate. It is an uncommon response to chronic *E. coli* infection. Malakoplakia appears as multiple mural filling defects secondary to submucosal granulomas.

c) **True** Leukoplakia also affects the ureter and collecting system. It is due to squamous metaplasia of transitional epithelium secondary to chronic infection or stones. It is believed to be a premalignant condition.

d) **True** However, emphysematous pyelonephritis more commonly results from Gram-negative infection in immunocompromised patients, including patients with diabetes mellitus. Nephrectomy is the treatment of choice. Emphysematous pyelonephritis is associated with a high mortality rate of up to 80%.

e) **True** Various genitourinary conditions occur in patients with AIDS, including HIV nephropathy, acute tubular necrosis, nephrocalcinosis, infection (such as cytomegalovirus, *Pneumocystis carinii* and *Mycobacterium avium-intracellulare* complex) and neoplasms (such as renal cell carcinoma, Kaposi's sarcoma, lymphoma, and testicular germ cell).

33 a) **False** The bladder neck commonly hypertrophies and appears narrowed compared with the dilated posterior urethra.

b) **True** The typical postinstrumentation stricture is short, well defined and lies in the bulbomembranous urethra. Infective strictures (most commonly due to *Neisseria gonorrhoeae*) result in a long beaded stricture in the bulbopenile region.

c) **False** The converse is true. Due to the attachment of the posterior urethra to the urogenital diaphragm, there is a high risk of a shearing injury to the urethra after a pelvic fracture (up to 15% in males with pelvic fractures, but less than 1% in females).

d) **False** Squamous cell carcinoma is the most common primary malignant tumour, but all urethral malignancies are rare. Adenocarcinoma is very rare and arises in Cowper's or Littré's glands. Stricture, trauma and infection are risk factors for squamous cell carcinoma.

e) **True** Acquired urethral diverticula result from infection of the paraurethral glands with subsequent rupture into the urethra. Complications include infection, calculi and adenocarcinoma.

34 a) **False** Recognised risk factors include: advancing age, testosterone (eunuchs almost never develop prostate adenocarcinoma), previous cadmium exposure and a diet high in animal fats.

b) **True** The level of this glycoprotein is elevated in 80% of cases of prostate cancer, but can also be raised by BPH and prostatitis. Cancers tend to elevate PSA levels much more than prostatic hypertrophy, which is the rationale behind calculating the PSA density (prostate volume divided by PSA level). Values of more than 0.12 are 90% sensitive for cancer.

c) **False** Although seminal vesical invasion is suggested by low signal that appears contiguous with the tumour, a similar appearance may be the result of post-biopsy change or amyloidosis.

d) **True** Other causes of hypoechoic lesions in the peripheral zone include atypical hyperplasia, focal prostatitis and prostatic cysts. On transrectal ultrasound, 30%–40% of prostate cancers are isoechoic to the normal prostate.

e) **False** Nodes measuring 10 mm or more in the short axis are considered to be abnormal.

35 a) **False** The routine use of contrast material is not necessary. Thin slice (3 mm) axial T2-weighted images are most useful.

b) **True** Thus, endorectal MRI studies are usually followed by axial T1-weighted imaging through the pelvis and lower abdomen to assess for nodal and bony spread.

c) **False** MRI spectroscopy evaluation of the relative signals of choline and citrate within the prostate gland has been found useful in the diagnosis of prostate cancer, particularly cancers arising in the central gland, in the evaluation of multicentric disease and also in distinguishing between postbiopsy change and tumour.

d) **True** Diagnostic uncertainty can occur when the peripheral zone is hypointense from fibrosis, BPH, postbiopsy haemorrhage or prostatitis.

e) **False** Several studies have shown that signs such as smooth capsular bulging, retraction or thickening are insufficiently accurate to predict capsular spread. Signs that are accurate in this regard are unequivocal extension into adjacent fat or neurovascular bundle, or invasion of the seminal vesicle.

36 a) **False** The epididymis is usually isoechoic or slightly hyperechoic to the testis.

b) **True** There is also an association of testicular microlithiasis with cryptorchidism, Down's syndrome, male pseudohermaphroditism and pulmonary alveolar microlithiasis. There is an increased incidence of germ cell tumour. On ultrasound, testicular microlithiasis appears as multiple (more than five per testicle) echogenic nonshadowing foci.

c) **True** In addition, epididymal cysts are seen in up to 40% of studies. Spermatocoeles are similar in appearance, but may contain internal low-level echoes.

d) **False** The epididymis is typically enlarged, hypervascular and hypoechoic. Coexisting orchitis is seen in 20% of cases and has a similar ultrasound appearance. Orchitis rarely occurs without associated epididymitis.

e) **False** In colour Doppler imaging of paediatric patients, intratesticular blood flow can be difficult to demonstrate. In one study (mean age 6.5 years), flow was absent bilaterally in 34% of cases and unilaterally in 8%. Power Doppler may be helpful in such cases.

37 a) **False** At term, 3.5% of testes are maldescended compared with 30% in premature babies. The testes are normally within the scrotum by 28–32 weeks' gestational age.

b) **True** Cryptorchidism is also associated with prune belly syndrome, Prader–Willi syndrome, Beckwith–Wiedemann syndrome and Lawrence–Moon–Biedl syndrome.

c) **True** MRI is probably the modality of choice in localising ectopic/maldescended testes. Ultrasonography is very sensitive when the testes lie within the inguinal region.

d) **True** There is also an increased risk of trauma, sterility and malignancy in cryptorchidism.

e) **False** Seminoma is the most common tumour in undescended testes. There is a 30–50-fold increased risk of testicular malignancy in cryptorchidism and the risk correlates with increasing distance from the scrotal sac. The risk is present even after orchiopexy.

38 a) **True** Recognised risk factors include: cryptorchidism, a personal or family history of testicular neoplasia, and Jewish or Caucasian race.

b) **False** Germ cell tumours account for 95% of testicular neoplasms. The remaining tumours are made up of sex cord-stromal tumours (Leydig's and Sertoli's cell tumours) and metastases.

c) **False** Seminoma is the most common germ cell tumour (40%–50%) and usually presents in the fourth to fifth decade of life. Teratomas occur at a younger age (during the second decade). Other germ cell tumours include embryonal cell carcinoma, choriocarcinoma (most aggressive), yolk sac tumour (most common germ cell tumour in infants, accounting for 60% of testicular neoplasms in this age group) and epidermoid cyst of the testicle (benign with possible 'onion skin' appearance). About 40% of tumours have mixed histology. On ultrasound, most tumours are hypoechoic (diagnosis of the exact tumour type requires histology).

d) **False** Choriocarcinomas are highly malignant tumours that metastasise early. Metastases may be present without evidence of choriocarcinoma in the testes.

e) **True** Lymphoma is the most common testicular neoplasm in men aged more than 50 years. In adults with metastatic disease to the testes, the primary sites include the prostate, lung, kidney, gastrointestinal tract, bladder, thyroid and melanoma. In children, primary sites include neuroblastoma, Wilms' tumour and rhabdomyosarcoma.

39 a) **False** There is a 10% incidence of malignancy in adrenal tumours, but this rate is higher for extra-adrenal tumours (up to 30%).

b) **True** About 10% of tumours are extra-adrenal (more than 30% in children) and they can lie anywhere from the neck to the pelvis; 2%–5% occur at the aortic bifurcation (organ of Zuckerkandl).

c) **True** There are numerous associations, including multiple endocrine neoplasia (types 2a and 2b), tuberous sclerosis, von Hippel–Lindau syndrome, NF and Carney syndrome.

d) **True** However, MIBG scintigraphy is still the most sensitive imaging test for extra-adrenal phaeochromocytoma.

e) **True** Although other adrenal neoplasms (eg, adrenal cortical carcinoma) can also be high signal on T2-weighted imaging, none of them are as hyperintense as phaeochromocytomas (lightbulb sign). The enhancement after gadolinium administration is most marked on the delayed (rather than the immediate) postcontrast images.

40 a) **True**   This is a rare tumour. It is more common than phaeochromocytoma.
It may occur at any age, but the peak incidence is between 30 and 50 years.

b) **True**   It is also associated with Beckwith–Wiedemann syndrome and astrocytomas.

c) **True**   The most common hormone produced in excess in adults is cortisol followed
by androgens, oestrogens and aldosterone.

d) **False**   Adrenal cortical carcinomas are bilateral in 10% of cases and slightly more
common on the left side. They are usually greater than 5 cm in size. On CT,
there is heterogeneous enhancement. The lesion is hyperintense to liver
on T2-weighted MRI.

e) **False**   Adrenal cortical carcinoma is normally resistant to radiotherapy. The prognosis
is generally poor.

Chapter 5

Musculoskeletal imaging

1 **Which of the following are true regarding congenital hypothyroidism?**
   a) It is more common in males
   b) The incidence is higher in infants with Down's syndrome
   c) A radiolucent metaphyseal band is a feature
   d) Sclerosis of the skull base occurs
   e) It is a cause of posterior scalloping of the vertebral bodies

2 **Cone-shaped epiphyses are seen in which of the following conditions?**
   a) Ellis–van Creveld syndrome
   b) Hypothyroidism
   c) Multiple epiphyseal dysplasia
   d) Achondroplasia
   e) Down's syndrome

3 **Which of the following statements are true regarding cleidocranial dysostosis?**
   a) It is inherited as an autosomal recessive trait
   b) Hypoplasia of the distal third of the clavicle is seen in the majority of cases
   c) It is associated with osteosclerosis
   d) It is associated with an absent radius and fibula
   e) Bladder exstrophy is a feature

4 **Which of the following statements are true regarding osteomalacia?**
   a) Looser's zones show increased uptake on radionuclide bone scan
   b) Looser's zones are most commonly seen along the medial border of the humeral neck
   c) There is an association with neurofibromatosis (NF)
   d) There is an association with melorheostosis
   e) It causes loss of the lamina dura of the teeth

5 **Which of the following are true regarding hyperparathyroidism?**
   a) Soft tissue calcifications are more common in secondary hyperparathyroidism
   b) Primary hyperparathyroidism is most commonly caused by parathyroid hyperplasia
   c) Secondary hyperparathyroidism results in a 'super scan' on radionuclide bone scan
   d) It is a cause of an erosive arthropathy
   e) It is a cause of cortical nephrocalcinosis

6 **Which of the following are true regarding lumbar discography?**
   a) Persistent low back pain at the L5/S1 level with a negative spinal magnetic resonance image is an appropriate indication
   b) It is usually performed via a transdural approach along the interspinous line
   c) To opacify the nucleus pulposus, 3 ml of contrast is usually required
   d) When combined with computed tomography (CT), it increases the sensitivity of detecting annular tear
   e) It is rarely performed because of the high risk of inducing disc herniation

7 **Which of the following statements are true?**
   a) Kienböck's disease is associated with a long ulna
   b) In the knee, osteochondritis dissecans occurs more frequently over the lateral femoral condyle
   c) Freiberg's disease is frequently bilateral
   d) Widening of the joint space is an early sign of Perthes disease
   e) Spontaneous osteonecrosis of the knee (SONK) frequently affects the medial femoral condyle

8 **Which of the following are true regarding Gorlin's syndrome?**
   a) It has a multifactorial aetiology
   b) Supernumerary teeth are a feature
   c) It is associated with dense calcification of the falx cerebri
   d) There is an increased incidence of cerebellar astrocytoma
   e) Block vertebrae are a feature

9 **Which of the following conditions are associated with thickening of the lamina dura of the teeth?**
   a) Cushing's syndrome
   b) Hypoparathyroidism
   c) Paget's disease
   d) Scleroderma
   e) Osteopetrosis

10 **Which of the following are true regarding Langerhans' cell histiocytosis?**
   a) Periosteal reaction is not a feature of bony involvement
   b) Lesions in the cranial vault typically show a bevelled edge
   c) Radionuclide bone scan is the most sensitive test to detect bony involvement
   d) Lesions within the long bones are typically metaphyseal
   e) It typically involves the vertebral body and posterior elements within the spine

11 **Which of the following are true regarding juvenile chronic arthritis?**
   a) Epiphyseal compression fracture occurs
   b) Wrist ankylosis is less common in juvenile chronic arthritis than in rheumatoid arthritis
   c) Joint space narrowing and erosions occur early in the disease
   d) It results in periostitis of the hands and feet
   e) Periarticular osteoporosis is a common finding

12 **Which of the following statements regarding multiple myeloma are true?**
   a) Skeletal radiographs are more sensitive than radionuclide bone scans in detecting bony lesions
   b) Skeletal radiographs are abnormal in the majority of patients at the time of presentation
   c) Sclerotic bone lesions are more commonly seen in POEMS (polyneuropathy, organomegaly, endocrinopathy, monoclonal gammopathy and skin changes) syndrome than in multiple myeloma
   d) Bony involvement typically spares the mandible
   e) Magnetic resonance imaging (MRI) of the lumbar spine is useful in the staging of patients with a normal skeletal survey

13 Which of the following are true regarding osteosarcoma?
a) There is an association with pineoblastoma
b) There is an increased incidence in osteopetrosis
c) Telangiectatic osteosarcoma typically demonstrates fluid-fluid levels on MRI
d) It frequently metastasises to other bones
e) Parosteal osteosarcoma resembles myositis ossificans on radiographs

14 Which of the following are true regarding soft tissue sarcomas?
a) Calcification is rarely seen in malignant fibrous histiocytoma
b) Myxoid liposarcoma appears near water density on CT
c) Synovial sarcomas show calcification in 30% of cases
d) Central necrosis is frequently seen in leiomyosarcoma
e) Malignant peripheral nerve sheath tumour is easily distinguished from neurofibroma on MRI

15 Extramedullary haemopoiesis occurs at which of the following sites?
a) Lymph nodes
b) Gastrointestinal tract
c) Thyroid gland
d) Spleen
e) Falx cerebri

16 Which of the following are true regarding ankylosing spondylitis?
a) It has an increased incidence in Afro-Caribbeans
d) Sacroiliitis is typically bilateral and symmetrical
c) It is associated with iritis in less than 5% of cases
d) It is a cause of atlanto-axial subluxation
e) There is an increased frequency of aortic stenosis

17 Which of the following are causes of atlanto-axial subluxation?
a) Ehlers–Danlos syndrome
b) Marfan's syndrome
c) Achondroplasia
d) Turner's syndrome
e) Psoriatic arthropathy

18 Which of the following statements are true regarding aneurysmal bone cysts?
a) They are more common in females
b) They may involve two contiguous vertebral bodies
c) There is an association with giant cell tumour
d) They do not show any tracer uptake on radionuclide bone scan
e) Patients are usually asymptomatic at presentation

19 Which of the following statements are true regarding congenital dislocation of the hips?
a) It is more common in females
b) There is an association with oligohydramnios
c) It is most commonly seen in first-born infants
d) It is usually bilateral
e) Premature osteoarthritis typically occurs between 10 and 20 years of age

20 Which of the following are true regarding Perthes disease?
a) Female gender is associated with a poorer prognosis
b) Bilateral hip involvement is more common in males
c) There is usually a family history
d) An older age of onset is associated with a better prognosis
e) It results in coxa magna

21 Which of the following MRI features are useful in distinguishing malignant from benign causes of vertebral collapse?
a) A convex posterior border of the collapsed vertebra
b) The presence of paravertebral soft tissue mass
c) A collapsed vertebral body showing low T1-weighted signal and high T2-weighted signal
d) The presence of spinal cord compression
e) A pattern of impaired diffusion on diffusion-weighted imaging

22 Which of the following statements are true?
a) Conversion of red marrow to yellow marrow proceeds from the axial to the peripheral skeleton
b) Reconversion of yellow marrow to red marrow proceeds from the axial to the peripheral skeleton
c) Infiltration of the marrow is best detected using a T2-weighted sequence
d) Chemical shift imaging is useful in detecting marrow infiltration
e) MRI abnormality in myelofibrosis is typically patchy in distribution

23 Which of the following are true regarding MRI of the knee?
a) MRI has a greater than 90% negative predictive value for meniscal tear
b) The double posterior cruciate ligament sign indicates a partial tear of the posterior cruciate ligament
c) On T2-weighted imaging, extension of the joint fluid between the medial meniscus and the joint capsule is a sign of meniscocapsular separation
d) Tear of the anterior cruciate ligament is frequently associated with contusion of the anterior lateral tibial plateau
e) Irregularity of the Hoffa's fat-pad is seen in rheumatoid arthritis

24 Which of the following statements are true regarding MRI arthrography of the shoulder?
a) 0.1 ml of gadopentetate dimeglumine (Gd-DTPA) diluted in 20 ml of normal saline is a suitable intra-articular contrast medium
b) The superior glenohumeral ligament is best identified on T1-weighted axial images at the level of the biceps tendon
c) Absence of the middle glenohumeral ligament is associated with absence of the anterosuperior labrum
d) The inferior glenohumeral ligament consists of an anterior and posterior band
e) MRI performed with the shoulder in abduction and external rotation improves the detection of labral tears

25 In MRI of the ankle and foot, which of the following are true?
  a) The posterior talofibular ligament is the most common ligament injured in ankle sprain
  b) The anterior talofibular ligament is best identified in the coronal plane
  c) Rupture of the Achilles tendon usually occurs at its insertion onto the calcaneum
  d) Tarsal tunnel syndrome is most commonly bilateral
  e) Morton's neuroma typically appears as a low-signal mass on both T1-weighted and T2-weighted imaging

26 Which of the following ultrasonographic signs may be seen in a full thickness rotator cuff tear of the shoulder?
  a) Nonvisualisation of the rotator cuff
  b) Full thickness focal hyperechogenicity of the rotator cuff
  c) Focal thinning of the rotator cuff
  d) Fluid in the subacromial-subdeltoid bursa
  e) Visualisation of the underlying hyaline cartilage

27 In MRI of the brachial plexus, which of the following are true?
  a) The middle trunk of the brachial plexus is formed exclusively by the C7 nerve root
  b) The cords of the brachial plexus are seen well on T1-weighted oblique sagittal images
  c) Radiation fibrosis typically appears low signal on T2-weighted images
  d) Intravenous gadolinium-DTPA is used to distinguish radiation fibrosis from malignant infiltration
  e) Heterogeneous signal on T2-weighted images favours the diagnosis of a malignant peripheral nerve sheath tumour over its benign counterpart

28 Which of the following statements are true regarding MRI of the wrist?
  a) The normal median nerve appears hyperintense to muscle on T2-weighted imaging
  b) The lunotriquetral and scapholunate ligaments are best demonstrated in the axial plane
  c) Tenosynovitis most frequently affects the extensor pollicis longus tendon
  d) The ulnar tunnel syndrome is frequently caused by a ganglion cyst
  e) Traumatic tears of the triangular fibrocartilage usually occur at the ulnar attachment

29 Which of the following are true regarding MRI of the elbow?
  a) MRI of the elbow is typically performed with the elbow held at 90° flexion
  b) The capitellum is a common site for osteochondritis dissecans of the elbow
  c) Rupture of the distal biceps tendon usually occurs at its insertion into the radius
  d) On axial images, the ulnar nerve is clearly seen within the cubital tunnel
  e) Following injection of steroid, increased signal intensity may be detected in the injected muscle or tendon on T2-weighted imaging for up to 1 month

30 Which of the following are the appropriate treatments for the conditions listed?
  a) Percutaneous vertebroplasty with polymethylmethacrylate (PMMA) for painful metastatic vertebral collapse
  b) Percutaneous discectomy for a sequestrated lumbar intervertebral disc
  c) Percutaneous removal of an osteoid osteoma with a bone biopsy needle
  d) Percutaneous injection of methylprednisolone acetate or Ethibloc for fibrous dysplasia
  e) Fluoroscopic-guided needle aspiration of calcific tendonitis of the shoulder

31 Which of the following statements regarding the spine are correct?
a) Osteoid osteoma is most commonly found within the vertebral body
b) Osteoblastoma is usually confined to the vertebral body
c) Giant cell tumour of the spine most frequently affects the sacrum
d) Aneurysmal bone cyst of the spine most frequently affects the sacrum
e) Chordoma of the sacrum does not cross the sacroiliac joint

32 Which of the following are true regarding musculoskeletal trauma?
a) Atlanto-occipital dislocation is frequently fatal
b) Sternal fracture is an indirect sign of thoracic spine injury
c) Laceration of the dura is commonly associated with lumbar spine fracture
d) A scapholunate angle of more than 80° is suggestive of scapholunate dissociation
e) Epiphyseal plate fractures (Salter–Harris type I) are common in nonaccidental injury in children

33 Which of the following are true in rheumatoid arthritis?
a) The arthritis is confined to synovial joints
b) The atlanto-axial joint is involved in 3% of cases
c) There is an increased risk of septic arthritis of the affected joint
d) Periostitis occurs in 20% of cases
e) Amyloidosis occurs as a complication in 20% of cases

34 Which of the following are true regarding pigmented villonodular synovitis?
a) It is five times more common in females
b) Soft tissue calcification is common
c) The knee is most frequently affected
d) Painful periarticular osteoporosis is an early feature
e) It causes well-defined bony erosions on both sides of an affected joint

35 Which of the following are true in the following conditions affecting the hands?
a) Subperiosteal bone resorption occurs in sarcoidosis
b) Sarcoidosis results in enlargement of the nutrient foramina of the phalanges
c) Tuberous sclerosis is associated with cystic lesions in the phalanges and metacarpals
d) Periarticular erosions occur early in systemic lupus erythematosus
e) Hypoplasia of the thumb is a feature of Down's syndrome

36 Which of the following are true regarding metastatic disease to the bones?
a) Medulloblastoma results in sclerotic metastases
b) Malignant melanoma is a cause of expansile metastases
c) The level of serum prostate-specific antigen (PSA) is typically normal in patients with metastatic prostate carcinoma
d) Retinoblastoma rarely metastasises to the bones
e) About 30% of colorectal carcinomas metastasise to the bones

37 Which of the following statements regarding the ribs are true?
a) Ribbon rib is a feature of NF
b) Short bulbous ribs occur in achondroplasia
c) Takayasu's arteritis results in superior rib notching
d) Fluorosis typically spares the ribs
e) Fibrous dysplasia of the ribs results in increased tracer uptake on radionuclide bone scan

38 **Which of the following are true of acro-osteolysis?**
   a) Frostbite typically affects the thumb
   b) Polyvinyl chloride exposure results in the resorption of the middle portion of the terminal phalanx
   c) It occurs in epileptics who are over-dosed with phenytoin
   d) It may result from dermatomyositis
   e) It may be caused by Lesch–Nyhan syndrome

39 **Which of the following statements are true?**
   a) Metaphyseal corner fracture is a feature of scurvy
   b) Metaphyseal corner fracture is a feature of nonaccidental injury in children
   c) Diaphyseal infarction occurs in thalassaemia
   d) Cubitus varus is a feature of Turner's syndrome
   e) Protrusio acetabuli occur in 40% of patients with Marfan's syndrome

40 **Which of the following are true regarding Erdheim–Chester disease?**
   a) Bony involvement is typically asymmetrical
   b) Bony sclerosis is a feature
   c) Infiltration of the perirenal space is common
   d) It is a cause of diabetes insipidus
   e) Unlike Langerhans' cell histiocytosis, the lung is not involved

Answers

1 a) **False** The condition is three times more common in females.
   b) **True**
   c) **False** The bones are slender, with endosteal thickening and typically with a dense band at the metaphysis.
   d) **True** Sclerosis at the skull base is a feature. Other skull changes include: brachycephaly, wormian bones, delayed fusion of the sutures and hypoplasia of the mastoid air cells and paranasal sinuses.
   e) **False** There may be hypoplasia of the vertebral bodies, particularly at the level of the first or second lumbar vertebrae (bullet-shaped). Posterior scalloping of the vertebral bodies is seen in acromegaly.

2 a) **True**
   b) **False**
   c) **True**
   d) **True**
   e) **False**

The causes of cone-shaped epiphysis include: dactylitis (sickle cell disease, frostbite, burns, osteomyelitis), trauma (battered child syndrome), congenital (achondroplasia, acrodysostosis, multiple epiphyseal dysplasia, Ellis–van Creveld syndrome, chondrodysplasia punctata), metabolic (hyperthyroidism in childhood) and those of idiopathic origin.

3 a) **False** The condition is inherited as an autosomal dominant trait. However, 33% of cases may arise from new mutations. Pyknodysostosis is inherited as an autosomal recessive trait.
   a) **False** Hypoplasia of the distal or middle third of the clavicle is encountered in 10% of cases.
   c) **False** Osteosclerosis is a feature of pyknodysostosis.
   d) **True** Other abnormalities of the appendicular skeleton include: elongated second metacarpals, short distal hand phalanges with pointed terminal tufts and accessory epiphyses in the hands and feet.
   e) **False** There is delayed ossification of the pubic bones, resulting in widening of the symphysis pubis. However, this does not result in full-blown bladder exstrophy.

4 a) **True** This is due to the increased bone turnover.
   b) **False** Looser's zones are most frequently found along the medial border of the femoral neck. Other common sites include the scapulae, the pubic rami, ribs, distal radii and proximal ulna.
   c) **True** Other associations include: melorheostosis, fibrous dysplasia, nonossifying fibroma, giant cell tumour and osteoblastoma.
   d) **True** See c).
   e) **True** Other metabolic causes include hyperparathyroidism and Cushing's syndrome.

5 a) **True** Secondary hyperparathyroidism usually results from chronic renal failure. Calcifications are frequently observed within the soft tissue and arterial wall.

b) **False** In 80%–90% of cases, primary hyperparathyroidism is due to a parathyroid adenoma. In 10%–15% of cases, it results from parathyroid hyperplasia. The degree of hypercalcaemia is related to the size of the adenoma. Ultrasonography has a diagnostic accuracy of up to 80% in the detection of parathyroid adenoma. However, radionuclide imaging with sestamibi also has a high diagnostic accuracy in detecting disease.

c) **True** 'Superscan' refers to an increased uptake of tracer within the bones, particularly within the axial skeleton, skull, costochondral junction, sternum and the long bones. There is an increased bone to soft tissue ratio and reduced activity within the kidneys. Common causes include: renal osteodystrophy, primary hyperparathyroidism, osteomalacia, diffuse skeletal metastases and myelofibrosis.

d) **True** Hyperparathyroidism results in marginal erosions, especially over the distal interphalangeal joint. The bones may demonstrate osteopenia with subperiosteal resorption and cortical tunnelling. It may be associated with chondrocalcinosis and periarticular soft tissue calcifications.

e) **False** Hyperparathyroidism may result in medullary nephrocalcinosis. Cortical nephrocalcinosis is most frequently seen in acute cortical necrosis, chronic glomerulonephritis and chronic transplant rejection. Other causes include Alport's syndrome, congenital oxalosis, methylene glycol poisoning and AIDS.

6 a) **True** Discography is an invasive test, which is reserved for patients who fail conservative treatment and where noninvasive diagnostic tests, such as magnetic resonance imaging (MRI), fail to yield diagnostic information. The indications for the test include negative MRI with recurrent and persistent symptoms, positive MRI with multiple levels of disc disease but uncertain symptomatic disc level, and recurrent symptoms following disc surgery. The test is positive if discogenic pain is reproduced by contrast injection.

b) **False** The procedure is normally performed with the patient prone and the needle inserted paramedially, 8 to 10 cm lateral to the midline, thus avoiding the dura.

c) **False** A normal disc takes up to 1–2 ml of contrast. Usually, 1 ml of nonionic contrast medium is adequate.

d) **True** CT following discography increases detection and grading of annular tears (radial, concentric and transverse).

e) **False** Discography does not injure the disc. However, there is a small risk (1%) of discitis following the procedure.

7 a) **False** Kienböck's disease (avascular necrosis of the lunate) is associated with a short ulna.

b) **False** Osteochondritis dissecans is more frequently seen over the lateral aspect of the medial femoral condyle. It is bilateral in up to 30% of cases.

c) **False** Freiberg's disease is typically unilateral and, unlike almost all other osteochondritides, is more common in females. It typically affects the head of the second metatarsal.

d) **True** Widening of the joint space (Waldenström sign) occurs early in Perthes disease.

e) **True** SONK typically occurs over the medial femoral condyle. It can also affect the medial tibial plateau.

8 a) **False** It has an autosomal dominant mode of inheritance.
     b) **True** The syndrome is characterised by multiple basal cell carcinomas and multiple jaw cysts (dentigerous cysts). Ectopic calcifications, such as that in the falx cerebri, are a feature. There is also an association with skeletal abnormalities, such as bifid ribs, block vertebrae, scoliosis and Sprengel's deformity of the scapula.
     c) **True**
     d) **False** The incidence of brain tumours is not increased, unlike in Turcot syndrome, which is the association of colonic polyposis with central nervous system tumours such as supratentorial glioblastoma.
     e) **True**

9 a) **False**
     b) **True**
     c) **False**
     d) **False**
     e) **True**

          Osteopetrosis and hypoparathyroidism are associated with thickening of the lamina dura of the teeth. Cushing's syndrome, Paget's disease and scleroderma cause loss of the lamina dura of the teeth, as do hyperparathyroidism, osteoporosis, osteomalacia, leukaemia, metastases and Langerhans' cell histiocytosis.

10 a) **False** Langerhans' cell histiocytosis results from an altered immune response. It affects children and young adults and is more common in males. Localised disease affecting a single bone is more common than disseminated disease. Long bones, the pelvis, vertebrae and the skull vault are common sites. A periosteal reaction may be seen.
     b) **True** Lesions in the skull typically have a bevelled edge, giving a 'hole-in-a-hole' or 'button sequestrum' appearance.
     c) **False** Radiographs are more sensitive than radionuclide bone scans, which may be negative in up to 35% of cases.
     d) **False** Lesions are usually diaphyseal, but may involve the epiphyses.
     e) **False** Langerhans' cell histiocytosis typically affects the vertebral bodies with sparing of the intervertebral discs and posterior elements. The collapse of a vertebral body results in 'vertebra plana'.

11 a) **True** Juvenile chronic arthritis occurs most frequently in children aged 1–5 years. Extra-articular manifestations are common and are frequently the presenting symptoms. The majority are negative for rheumatoid factor. The disease can result in overgrowth or undergrowth of the epiphyses and epiphyseal compression fractures.
     b) **False** Bony ankylosis frequently affects the carpal and tarsal bones in juvenile chronic arthritis. Ankylosis is less frequently encountered in rheumatoid arthritis.
     c) **False** Unlike rheumatoid arthritis, where joint space narrowing and bony erosions occur early, these features tend to occur late in juvenile chronic arthritis.
     d) **True** Periarticular periostitis is common, especially affecting the phalanges.
     e) **True**

12 a) **True**   Technetium-99m diphosphonate bone scans are usually normal or show diminished uptake. Bone scintigraphy is insensitive in the detection of bone lesions, especially in the skull.

b) **True**   About 80% of patients have abnormal radiographs at presentation. The range of abnormality includes osteopenia, sharply defined focal bone lucencies, vertebral collapse, expansile bone lesions, permeative change and sclerotic foci (2%). Sites of involvement include vertebrae (66%), ribs (45%), skull (40%), shoulder (40%), pelvis (30%) and the long bones (25%).

c) **True**   POEMS syndrome is a rare multisystem disorder of obscure pathogenesis characterised by polyneuropathy, organomegaly, endocrinopathy of various forms, production of a monoclonal component and skin changes. This syndrome occurs in only about 1% of plasmacytoma cases, but in more than 50% of the rare osteosclerotic subtypes and plasma cell dyscrasias.

d) **False**   Unlike bony metastases, which rarely affect the mandible, involvement of the mandible is not unusual in myeloma.

e) **True**   MRI of the spine shows abnormality in 50% of patients with normal radiographs. Some centres now routinely use MRI in the staging of myeloma. Patients with marrow infiltrates on MRI have an increased risk of early disease progression. MRI is also the imaging modality of choice for suspected epidural involvement and for the assessment of the response of vertebral lesions to treatment.

13 a) **True**   There is an association with bilateral retinoblastoma and pineoblastoma.

b) **True**   The incidence is increased in patients with osteopetrosis, Paget's disease and prior radiotherapy. The peak incidence is at age 15–20 years. About 75% of cases arise in the metaphyseal region of the distal femur or proximal tibia.

c) **True**   Telangiectatic osteosarcomas (5%) are aggressive high-grade tumours with little osteoid formation in the matrix, and hence appear completely osteolytic. Pathological fractures are common. Fluid-fluid levels are typically seen on CT or MRI.

d) **False**   Metastatic spread is haematogenous, as bones lack a lymphatic system. The lungs are the most frequent sites, although bones may be involved. Lymphadenopathy occurs late in the disease and is a poor prognostic sign.

e) **True**   Parosteal osteosarcoma accounts for 4%–5% of all osteosarcomas. They develop in the cortex of the bone, sparing the medulla, and grow circumferentially around the bone. They are low-grade lesions and have the best prognosis. The appearance may resemble myositis ossificans, although the presence of peripheral calcifications in the mass and a clear plane of separation from the underlying bone favour the latter.

14 a) **False** Malignant fibrous histiocytoma is the most common soft tissue sarcoma (24% of cases), occurring in the extremities, craniofacial region and the retroperitoneum. Three main histological subtypes exist: storiform/pleomorphic (most common), myxoid and inflammatory. Coarse calcifications occur in up to 16% of cases, usually in the storiform/pleomorphic subtype.

   b) **True** Liposarcoma occurs most frequently between 40 and 60 years of age. Five main histological subtypes are recognised: well-differentiated, myxoid, round-cell, pleomorphic and de-differentiated. Myxoid liposarcomas contain gelatinous material and consequently may appear cystic and near water density on CT. Well-differentiated tumours typically contain visible fat.

   c) **True** Synovial sarcomas affect adults aged 20–40 years. Although they tend to arise near a joint, bursa or tendon sheath, the tissue of origin is not synovium but undifferentiated mesenchyme. About 30% contain calcifications, which denote a more favourable prognosis. Haemorrhage may be present in up to 40% and a fluid–fluid level in 20% of cases. Unlike many soft tissue sarcomas, nodal spread is common and is observed in up to 20% of cases at diagnosis.

   d) **True** Leiomyosarcomas frequently appear heterogeneous with a central necrosis. About 40% of patients have metastases at the time of diagnosis. Three patterns of growth have been described: completely extravascular, completely intravascular, and mixed extravascular and intravascular.

   e) **False** Although a large size (greater than 5 cm), loss of the target sign on T2-weighted MRI and irregularity suggest a malignant tumour, differentiation from benign neurofibroma is difficult. Malignant peripheral nerve sheath tumours are high-grade tumours, which frequently metastasise (65% of cases) and have a propensity to recur following resection.

15 All true Extramedullary haemopoiesis occurs when there is diminished or abnormal marrow haemopoietic activity. This occurs in various haematological conditions, such as thalassaemia, sickle cell anaemia and myelofibrosis. Extramedullary haemopoiesis occurs in a variety of sites including the lymph nodes, spleen, gastrointestinal tract and falx cerebri.

16 a) **False** The condition is most common in Caucasians. The incidence is three-fold greater in men than in women and 95% of patients are HLA B27 positive.

   b) **True** The axial skeleton is involved in most cases. Sacroiliitis is typically bilateral and symmetrical. Involvement of the appendicular skeleton is less common (10%–20% of cases). The temporomandibular joint may rarely be affected.

   c) **False** Iritis occurs in up to 25% of patients and is more frequently encountered in those with a peripheral arthropathy.

   d) **True** Atlanto-axial subluxation may result due to laxity of the transverse ligament from synovitis.

   e) **False** There is an increased incidence of aortic incompetence (5%) due to aortitis. About 1% of patients develop bilateral upper lobe pulmonary fibrosis.

17 a) **False**
   b) **True**
   c) **False**
   d) **False**
   e) **True**

Apart from trauma and infection, the two main groups of causes are congenital and the arthritides. Congenital causes include: Down's syndrome, Marfan's syndrome, Morquio's disease, spondyloepiphyseal dysplasia, chondrodysplasia punctata and pseudoachondroplasia. Arthritic causes include: rheumatoid arthritis, juvenile chronic arthritis, psoriatic arthritis, ankylosing spondylitis, systemic lupus erythematosus, gout/pseudogout, Reiter's syndrome (rare) and Behçet's syndrome (rare).

18 a) **True**   Aneurysmal bone cysts occur in growing bones in patients aged 10 to 30 years and are more common in females.
   b) **True**   Lesions occur in the unfused metaphysis of long bones, or in the metaphysis and epiphysis of bones after fusion; 20%–30% occur within the spine and up to 25% affect two contiguous vertebral bodies. Lesions are typically expansile and the thin but intact cortex may be difficult to discern. On CT, fluid–fluid levels are typically seen within the lesion.
   c) **True**   Up to one third of cases are associated with an underlying bone abnormality, such as a giant cell tumour.
   d) **False** Aneurysmal bone cysts show increased blood pooling activity on bone scintigraphy.
   e) **False** Patients are usually symptomatic at presentation, complaining of pain and swelling.

19 a) **True**   Congenital dislocation of the hips is eight times more common in females. It is most common amongst Caucasians.
   b) **True**   Oligohydramnios is a risk factor. Other risk factors include breech presentation, a prior family history, foot deformities, skull-moulding deformities and congenital torticollis.
   c) **True**   Two thirds of cases occur in the firstborn child.
   d) **False** Two thirds of cases are unilateral. The left side is more frequently affected than the right.
   e) **False** Secondary osteoarthritis is typically not apparent until 40–60 years of age.

20 a) **True**   Females have an earlier onset of disease, but a poorer prognosis. However, the disease is more common in males.
   b) **True**   Bilateral disease is more common in males. However, involvement is rarely synchronous or symmetrical.
   c) **False** There is no increased incidence in families. However, there is reportedly an associated increased incidence of cardiac abnormality, pyloric stenosis, renal abnormality and undescended testes.
   d) **False** Poor prognostic factors include the female sex, an older onset of disease, metaphyseal involvement, a greater degree of epiphyseal involvement (Caterell's grade III or VI) and uncovering of the lateral femoral neck.
   e) **True**   Coxa magna is a late sequela of the disease and is typified by a remodelled femoral head, which is wider and flatter with a mushroom configuration.

21 a) **True**   A convex posterior border suggests underlying vertebral infiltration, especially when associated with epidural compression. Other signs in favour of metastatic infiltration include complete replacement of marrow signal in the vertebral body and extension of abnormal signal into the pedicles/posterior elements.

    b) **True**

    c) **False**   Both osteoporotic and metastatic vertebral body fractures can result in high T2-weighted and low T1-weighted signal acutely. Follow-up MRI 6 weeks after trauma may be useful to look for a return towards normal marrow signal within the vertebra, which would suggest a benign aetiology.

    d) **False**   The presence of cord compression alone does not necessarily indicate a malignant cause.

    e) **True**   Tumour infiltration typically causes a greater limitation in diffusion compared with osteoporotic collapse.

22 a) **False**   From early childhood, the conversion of red to yellow marrow proceeds rapidly, beginning with the peripheral appendicular skeleton and progressing centrally. In adults, red marrow is normally localised to the axial skeleton and proximal femora and humeri.

    b) **True**   Marrow reconversion proceeds from the axial to the appendicular skeleton.

    c) **False**   Marrow infiltration is usually best detected on T1-weighted images, as the low signal infiltrates are easily discernible against the high signal of the fatty marrow.

    d) **True**   In-phase and out-of-phase imaging may be helpful in distinguishing an area of marrow infiltration from normal fat-containing marrow.

    e) **True**   Myelofibrosis typically affects the marrow in a widespread but patchy distribution.

23 a) **True**   Several large MRI studies have found the negative predictive value greater than 90% for meniscal tear. MRI has a slightly higher sensitivity and specificity for medial compared with lateral meniscal tear.

    b) **False**   A bucket-handle tear of the medial meniscus results in the double posterior cruciate ligament sign due to medial displacement of the meniscal fragment.

    c) **True**   Meniscocapsular separation may be suggested when this is seen within the medial joint compartment. However, this is not necessarily true when the same is observed in the lateral compartment of the knee. The diagnosis is best made on arthroscopy.

    d) **False**   The classic bone-bruising pattern results from anterior subluxation of the tibia. There is marrow oedema within the anterior aspect of the lateral femoral condyle immediately adjacent to the anterior horn of the lateral meniscus and in the posterolateral tibial plateau. There is frequently an associated medial meniscal tear.

    e) **True**   Irregularity of the Hoffa's fat pad is an early sign of synovitis in rheumatoid arthritis.

24 a) **True** MRI arthrography is increasingly used to evaluate shoulder instability. Typically, 10–12 ml of contrast containing Gd-DTPA in a dilution of 1:200 is administered intra-articularly under fluoroscopic guidance.

b) **True** The superior glenohumeral ligament comprises bands of thickened joint capsule and is the most consistently identified capsular ligament. It can arise from the anterosuperior labrum, the attachment of the long head of the biceps tendon or even the middle glenohumeral ligament. It is best seen on axial images, at or just above the level of the long head of the biceps tendon.

c) **False** Absence of the anterosuperior labrum is associated with cord-like thickening of the middle glenohumeral ligament (Bufford complex). It occurs in 1.5% of individuals.

d) **True** The inferior glenohumeral ligament consists of an anterior and posterior band, with the axillary recess lying between the two.

e) **True** MRI with the shoulder in abduction and external rotation (ABER position) improves the detection of anterior labral tears and superior labral anterior–posterior (SLAP) lesions.

25 a) **False** The anterior talofibular ligament is the most common ligament injured, followed by the calcaneofibular ligament, then the posterior talofibular ligament.

b) **False** The anterior talofibular ligament is best visualised on axial images.

c) **False** Rupture of the Achilles tendon usually occurs 2–6 cm above its insertion onto the calcaneum. Rupture of the tendon at its insertion is uncommon and is associated with Haglund's deformity (prominent posterosuperior calcaneal tuberosity).

d) **False** Unlike carpal tunnel syndrome, this condition is usually unilateral.

e) **True** Morton's neuroma arises from a plantar digital nerve. It is more common in females, frequently located between the heads of the third and fourth metatarsals. The mass typically appears low-to-intermediate signal on both T1-weighted and T2-weighted imaging, attributed to the presence of fibrous tissue. Mild but variable enhancement occurs following intravenous gadolinium.

26 a) **True**

b) **False**

c) **True**

d) **True**

e) **True**

The ultrasonographic signs of a full thickness rotator cuff tear include non-visualisation or absence of the cuff tissue, a full thickness hypoechoic defect, focal thinning in the cuff, fluid in the subacromial-subdeltoid bursa, loss of the normal convexity of the cuff contour, exposure and visualisation of the underlying hyaline cartilage, and the ability to compress the deltoid muscle against the humeral head.

27 a) **True** The roots of the brachial plexus are derived from the anterior divisions of the spinal nerves of C5 to T1. The C5 and C6 roots combine to form the upper trunk, the C8 and T1 roots form the lower trunk and the middle trunk is derived from the C7 root. The three cords (lateral, medial and posterior) are derived from the anterior and posterior divisions of the trunks.

b) **True** The brachial plexus is well seen on axial and coronal images, but the cords are best demonstrated in relation to the subclavian artery in the oblique sagittal plane.

c) **True** Radiation fibrosis appears as diffuse thickening and enhancement of the brachial plexus without a focal mass. The soft tissue abnormality typically appears low signal on both T1-weighted and T2-weighted images.

d) **False** Both radiation fibrosis and tumour infiltration can show enhancement following intravenous gadolinium-DTPA. The presence of a mass that is low signal on T1-weighted and high signal on T2-weighted images is more suggestive of a tumour.

e) **True** There is overlap in the MRI features of benign and malignant neural tumours. Findings in favour of a malignant tumour include a large size (greater than 5 cm), irregular margins and internal heterogeneity.

28 a) **True** The normal median nerve appears hyperintense to muscle. Hence, the diagnosis of carpal tunnel syndrome should be made on a combination of signs: enlargement of the nerve proximal to the transverse carpal ligament, flattening of the median nerve, increased signal intensity and volar bulging of the flexor retinaculum.

b) **False** These ligaments are best visualised in the coronal planes. The ulnolunate, lunate and ulnotriquetral ligaments, although not consistently seen, are best visualised on sagittal images.

c) **False** Tenosynovitis usually affects the tendons of the flexor carpi ulnaris, flexor carpi radialis, abductor pollicis longus and extensor pollicis brevis (de Quervain's disease) muscles, and also the tendon of extensor carpi ulnaris.

d) **True** The ulnar tunnel (Guyon's tunnel), which transmits the ulnar artery and nerve, lies superficial to the flexor retinaculum, closely related to the hook of hamate bone and the pisiform bone. A ganglion cyst within the ulnar tunnel usually causes ulnar nerve impingement.

e) **False** Unlike degenerative tears, traumatic tears of the triangular fibrocartilage frequently occur within 1–2 mm of its radial attachment.

29 a) **False** The elbow is typically imaged with the patient supine with the arm at the side. The prone position may be adopted with the arm extended overhead.

b) **True** Osteochondritis dissecans most commonly affects the capitellum within the elbow. The anterior capitellum is frequently involved and should be distinguished from the pseudodefect (normal finding) that occurs posterolaterally. MRI is useful for staging of the abnormality.

c) **True** Rupture of the distal biceps tendon is more common in men. Complete rupture of the tendon from its insertion on the radial tuberosity is most common.

d) **True** The ulnar nerve is well seen on axial MRI as it courses through the cubital tunnel. The roof of the tunnel is formed by the cubital tunnel retinaculum. Thickening of the retinaculum results in entrapment of the nerve during elbow flexion. MRI features of neuritis and entrapment include swelling and enlargement of the proximal nerve and increased T2-weighted signal.

e) **True** Hence, MRI of the elbow should be performed prior to any intra-articular or periarticular steroid injections.

30 a) **True** Percutaneous vertebroplasty may be performed using PMMA for vertebral haemangiomas, or malignant or osteoporotic vertebral collapse. Injection of this cement material stabilises the spine leading to alleviation of pain.

b) **False** Percutaneous lumbar discectomy can be performed in patients whose disc herniations are contained behind the annulus or the posterior longitudinal ligament. The likelihood of success with a sequestrated disc is low.

c) **True** Ablation of an osteoid osteoma can be successfully achieved by removal of the central nidus with a trephine biopsy needle under CT guidance.

d) **False** Intra-osseous injection of methylprednisolone acetate may be used in the treatment of simple bone cysts. Injection of Ethibloc can be utilised in the treatment of both simple and aneurysmal bone cysts.

e) **True** Removal of the hydroxyapatite crystals can improve the night pain experienced by these patients. Aspiration of the calcium deposit is usually followed with an *in situ* injection of corticosteroid.

31 a) **False** The majority of osteoid osteomas in the spine (75% of cases) are located within the posterior elements (pedicles, articular facets and laminae). Only 7% are within vertebral bodies. Patients present with a painful scoliosis, with the pain typically being worst at night and relieved by salicylates.

b) **False** Osteoblastoma affects the posterior elements in 55% of cases, with extension into the vertebral body in 45% of cases. However, isolated involvement of the vertebral body is rare. Unlike osteoid osteoma, the pain produced by osteoblastoma is usually dull and may be associated with neurological symptoms, such as paraesthesia and paraparesis.

c) **True** The sacrum is the most common site of involvement followed by the vertebral bodies of the thoracic, cervical and lumbar spine. There is usually bony expansion. In the sacrum, extension across the sacroiliac joint is not unusual.

d) **False** The thoracic spine is the most common site of involvement, followed by the lumbar and cervical segments. Involvement of the sacrum is rare.

e) **False** Chordoma of the sacrum presents as a destructive lesion, usually at the level of S4 or S5, centred on the midline, without bony expansion, and associated with a soft tissue mass that frequently calcifies. The tumour can sometimes cross the intervertebral disc space or the sacroiliac joint.

32 a) **True** Atlanto-occipital dislocation is usually a fatal injury. The diagnosis is frequently missed and CT is frequently needed to make a confident diagnosis. Nevertheless, the diagnosis should be suspected in traumatised patients with findings of brainstem injury.

b) **True** A severe axial load to the upper thoracic spine can result in a fracture of the sternum, with posterior displacement of the upper fracture fragment. This pattern of injury is called an indirect sternal fracture and is associated with thoracic spine injury. Fractures of posterolateral and posteromedial ribs, with or without associated costovertebral dislocation, are also indirect signs of thoracic spinal injury.

c) **False** This is uncommon, occurring in 7%–16% of cases. It is more common in patients with a burst fracture that is associated with neurological deficit and laminae fracture.

d) **True** The normal scapholunate angle measures 30°–60°. Disruption of the scapholunate angle allows the scaphoid to rotate volar and the lunate dorsal resulting in widening of the angle (greater than 80°). This is also seen in dorsal intercalated segmental instability (DISI). Values less than 30° are seen in ventral intercalated segmental instability (VISI).

e) **False** Epiphyseal plate injuries are rarely encountered in nonaccidental trauma.

33 a) **False** Although the disease predominantly affects the synovial joints, cartilaginous joints such as the symphysis pubis and manubriosternal joint may also be involved.

b) **False** The atlanto-axial joint is commonly affected in up to 25% of cases.

c) **True** The inflamed joints are at increased risk of developing septic arthritis.

d) **False** Periostitis and periosteal reaction is unusual, occurring in less than 5% of cases.

e) **False** Amyloidosis is an uncommon complication.

34 a) **False** There is an equal incidence in males and females.

b) **False** Calcification is not a feature until late in the disease, although the periarticular soft tissue may appear dense because of haemosiderin deposition. Unlike pigmented villonodular synovitis, synovial sarcoma frequently exhibits calcifications (33% of cases) and appears high signal on T2-weighted MRI.

c) **True** Monoarticular involvement is usual (75% of cases), with the knee being most frequently affected.

d) **False** Periarticular osteoporosis is unusual, but may occur late in the disease.

e) **True** Pigmented villonodular synovitis causes well-defined erosions on either side of the affected joint, often with sclerotic borders.

35 a) **True** Subperiosteal resorption of bone may occur in sarcoidosis, mimicking hyperparathyroidism.

b) **True** Enlargement of the nutrient foramina is a feature of sarcoidosis.

c) **True** Patchy areas of bony sclerosis may also be observed.

d) **False** Bilateral symmetrical arthritis occurs. Soft tissue swelling and periarticular osteoporosis is common, but not periarticular erosions, which occur late in the disease.

e) **False** Hypoplasia of the middle phalanx of the little finger occurs in Down's syndrome. A short thumb occurs in myositis ossificans progressiva, Fanconi's anaemia and Holt–Oram syndrome.

36 a) **True** Sclerotic bone metastases commonly result from carcinoma of the prostate, breast, colon and stomach, lymphoma and carcinoid, and less frequently from other tumours, such as lung, bladder, myeloma and pancreas.

b) **True** Expansile metastases are typically observed with renal cell and thyroid carcinoma, phaeochromocytoma, myeloma and breast and bronchogenic carcinoma.

c) **False** The serum PSA and alkaline phosphatase levels are usually elevated.

d) **False** Retinoblastoma is a well-recognised cause of bone metastasis, especially in children.

e) **False** Less than 5% of colorectal carcinoma results in bony metastases.

37 a) **True** Ribbon ribs are most frequently seen in NF and osteogenesis imperfecta.

b) **True** Short bulbous ribs ('paddle-like' ribs) are typical of achondroplasia.

c) **False** Takayasu's arteritis results in inferior rib notching due to dilatation of the intercostal arteries.

d) **False** Fluorosis, myelofibrosis, mastocytosis and osteopetrosis result in sclerotic ribs.

e) **True** Fibrous dysplasia shows tracer uptake on radionuclide bone scan. Rib involvement occurs in 30% of patients with fibrous dysplasia.

38 a) **False** Frostbite typically spares the thumb.

b) **True**

c) **False** Acro-osteolysis may occur congenitally in infants of epileptic mothers with phenytoin toxicity.

d) **True** It may also result from other collagen vascular diseases, such as scleroderma, systemic lupus erythematosus and Sjögren's syndrome.

e) **True** It may be caused by Lesch–Nyhan syndrome as a result of repeated trauma from self-mutilation.

39 a) **True** Metaphyseal corner fracture may be seen in scurvy and nonaccidental injuries.

b) **True** Metaphyseal corner fracture results from a sudden twisting motion and is seen in about 10% of cases of nonaccidental injuries. It is most common around the knee, elbow, distal forearm and leg.

c) **False** Diaphyseal infarction occurs in sickle cell anaemia, but not thalassaemia.

d) **False** Cubitus valgus, but not cubitus varus, occurs in 60%–70% of patients with Turner's syndrome.

e) **True** Protrusio acetabuli is common in patients with Marfan's syndrome, occurring in 40% of cases.

40 a) **False**
  b) **True**
  c) **True**
  d) **True**
  e) **False**

Erdheim–Chester disease is a xanthogranulomatous infiltrative disease of unknown aetiology, with multisystemic involvement. Long bones (lower limbs more than upper limbs) are typically affected in the skeletal system, and involvement is usually symmetrical. There is usually sclerosis within the diaphyses or metaphyses associated with cortical thickening or coarsening of the trabeculae. There is usually sparing of the epiphyses and the axial skeleton. The retroperitoneum and the kidney are frequently involved. Involvement of the central nervous system results in diabetes insipidus, cerebellar symptoms and orbital lesions. Pulmonary involvement occurs in 20% of cases, resulting in upper lobe fibrosis. Pericardial effusion and hepatosplenomegaly can also occur.

Chapter 6

Neuroradiology

1 **Regarding the normal central nervous system, which of the following are true?**
   a) The corpus callosum develops from the posterior to the anterior
   b) The bones of the skull vault develop via intramembranous ossification
   c) The conus is normally located at L2/3 at birth
   d) On magnetic resonance imaging (MRI), the posterior lobe of the pituitary is hyperintense on T1-weighted imaging
   e) A cavum septi pellucidi (CSP) is present in 5%–15% of adults

2 **Which of the following are true concerning ultrasound of the central nervous system (CNS)?**
   a) The biparietal diameter is measured in an axial plane at the level of the thalami
   b) The normal cisterna magna is visualised in more than 90% of second trimester foetuses
   c) Anencephaly should be identifiable in more than 95% of cases by 14 weeks gestational age
   d) Choroid plexus cysts are seen in 20% of antenatal ultrasound scans
   e) Acute subependymal germinal matrix haemorrhage appears hypoechoic

3 **Concerning neuronal migration disorders, which of the following are true?**
   a) In schizencephaly the cleft is lined by mature white matter
   b) The septum pellucidum is absent in 90% of cases of schizencephaly
   c) Agyria–pachygyria is seen in Zellweger syndrome
   d) Nodular heterotopias do not enhance and are isointense to cortical grey matter
   e) Polymicrogyria is most common around the sylvian fissure

4 **Which of the following are true of holoprosencephaly?**
   a) It results from absence of the supraclinoid internal carotid artery (ICA) system
   b) Trisomy 13 is the most common associated chromosomal abnormality
   c) The septum pellucidum can be seen in the lobar subtype
   d) The falx cerebri may be seen anteriorly in the semilobar type
   e) The cerebellum is structurally normal in the alobar type

5 **Regarding the Dandy–Walker malformation, which of the following are true?**
   a) The posterior fossa is abnormally small
   b) The floor of the fourth ventricle is present
   c) The vermian remnant is inferiorly displaced
   d) Obstructive hydrocephalus occurs in about 80% of cases
   e) There is an association with polydactyly

6 **Regarding Chiari malformations, which of the following are true?**
   a) The Chiari I malformation is associated with myelomeningoceles
   b) In the Chiari II malformation, the fourth ventricle has an increased antero-posterior diameter
   c) The foramen magnum is typically small in the Chiari II malformation
   d) The lacunar skull changes of the Chiari II malformation tend to diminish with age
   e) Encephalocoeles are always present in the Chiari III malformation

7 **Concerning the Sturge–Weber syndrome, which of the following are true?**
   a) The inheritance is autosomal dominant
   b) The cutaneous lesion is most common in the distribution of the ophthalmic nerve
   c) The cortical abnormalities are usually contralateral to the cutaneous lesion
   d) Ipsilateral choroid plexus atrophy is common
   e) It is associated with Klippel–Trenaunay syndrome

8 **Which of the following are true of central (type 2) neurofibromatosis (NF-2)?**
   a) The inherited cases are usually due to a defect on chromosome 17
   b) Bilateral acoustic schwannomas alone allow a definite diagnosis of NF-2
   c) The trigeminal nerve is the next most commonly involved nerve after the eighth cranial nerve
   d) There is an increased incidence of optic nerve gliomas
   e) The most common spinal intramedullary tumour is an ependymoma

9 **In tuberous sclerosis affecting the brain, which of the following are true?**
   a) Cortical tubers undergo neoplastic change
   b) Cortical tubers enhance avidly
   c) Giant cell astrocytomas develop in approximately 15% of cases
   d) In adults, the heterotopic grey matter islands are hypointense on T2-weighted images
   e) Subependymal nodules are seen in fewer than 50% of cases

10 **Regarding colloid cysts of the third ventricle, which of the following are true?**
   a) They are usually present in childhood
   b) They typically arise adjacent to the sylvian aqueduct
   c) They are usually hypodense on unenhanced computed tomography (CT)
   d) They centrally enhance after intravenous iodinated contrast medium
   e) On T2-weighted MRI, they are typically hyperintense

11 **Regarding arachnoid cysts and epidermoid cysts, which of the following are true?**
   a) The cerebellopontine angle (CPA) is the most common location for arachnoid cysts
   b) The CPA is the most common location for epidermoid cysts
   c) Arachnoid cysts are classically isointense to cerebrospinal fluid (CSF) on all MRI sequences
   d) Epidermoid cysts typically encase and engulf arteries and cranial nerves
   e) Calcification is more common in epidermoid cysts

12 **Regarding glioblastoma multiforme, which of the following are true?**
   a) It is the most common primary brain tumour
   b) It has a peak incidence in the third and fourth decades
   c) It is associated with NF-1
   d) It is most commonly located in the grey matter of the cerebral hemispheres
   e) Classically, there is little peritumoural oedema

13 **Regarding pituitary adenomas, which of the following are true?**
   a) Macroadenomas are defined as those causing mass effect
   b) Adrenocorticotrophic hormone (ACTH)-secreting tumours are the most common type of pituitary microadenoma
   c) They calcify in less than 10% of cases
   d) Microadenomas typically enhance more than the normal pituitary
   e) They are histologically benign in more than 95% of cases

14 **Which of the following are true regarding craniopharyngioma?**
   a) They are most common in the fifth and sixth decades of life
   b) About 15% are malignant
   c) Craniopharyngiomas are purely intrasellar in about 10% of cases
   d) Visualisation of calcification makes the diagnosis unlikely
   e) They are usually hyperintense on T2-weighted imaging

15 **Concerning intracranial meningiomas, which of the following are true?**
   a) They are associated with NF-2
   b) The intraventricular type is more common in children than adults
   c) On CT, they are typically hyperdense and nonenhancing
   d) On MRI, a dural tail is seen in 90% of cases
   e) They are more likely to be benign if they give a high signal on T2-weighted imaging

16 **Concerning medulloblastoma, which of the following are true?**
   a) There is an association with Gorlin's syndrome
   b) About 75% of tumours occur in the first decade of life
   c) They are more frequently midline in location in adults than in children
   d) They are typically cystic, with an enhancing mural nodule
   e) The liver is the most common metastatic site outside of the nervous system

17 **Regarding acoustic neuromas, which of the following are true?**
   a) They most commonly originate from the cochlear division of the VIII nerve
   b) Bilateral tumours are diagnostic of NF-1
   c) They are usually isodense on unenhanced CT
   d) On T2-weighted imaging, they are hyperintense and enhance avidly after gadolinium administration
   e) Approximately 10%–30% show some degree of calcification on CT

18 **Concerning intracranial metastases, which of the following are true?**
   a) In most series they account for more than 40% of intracranial tumours
   b) They are most commonly located at the junction of the grey and white matter
   c) About 75% of metastatic lesions are single when initially detected on imaging
   d) Metastases from sarcomas are rare
   e) Small cell lung cancer metastasis within the medial temporal lobe is the most common cause of limbic encephalitis

19 Calcification of the basal ganglia is a recognised finding in which of the following?
a) Hypoparathyroidism
b) Hypothyroidism
c) AIDS
d) Fahr's disease
e) Cockayne's syndrome

20 Which of the following are true of the basal ganglia?
a) The lentiform nucleus consists of the lateral putamen and medial globus pallidus
b) Copper deposition in Wilson's disease typically causes high-density basal ganglia
c) Low attenuation basal ganglia are seen in hypoglycaemia
d) On T1-weighted imaging, hyperintense basal ganglia are seen in NF
e) On T2-weighted imaging, hypointense basal ganglia are seen in multiple sclerosis

21 Regarding granulomatous disease of the CNS, which of the following are true?
a) The most common CNS manifestation of tuberculosis is a tuberculoma
b) In adults, tuberculomas occur most commonly in the cerebral hemispheres and basal ganglia
c) Clinical involvement of the CNS occurs in less than 10% of patients with sarcoidosis
d) Granulomatous meningitis is seen in coccidioidomycosis
e) Granulomatous angiitis preferentially affects small vessels

22 Which of the following are true of herpes simplex encephalitis (HSE)?
a) It is the most common nonepidemic cause of viral encephalitis
b) In neonates, it is usually caused by herpes simplex virus type 2 (HSV-2)
c) Adult infection classically affects the limbic system bilaterally and symmetrically
d) The basal ganglia tend to be spared in adult HSE
e) Enhancement on CT persisting beyond 28 days indicates treatment failure

23 Concerning the neuroimaging of patients with AIDS, which of the following are true?
a) HIV encephalopathy (HIVE) results from an opportunistic infection
b) The imaging findings in HIVE may improve after protease inhibitor treatment
c) Progressive multifocal encephalopathy (PML) spares subcortical white matter
d) Toxoplasmosis is more likely than lymphoma if the lesions are multifocal
e) Basal ganglia involvement in cryptococcosis is unusual

24 Which of the following are true of multiple sclerosis?
a) Infratentorial plaques are more common in children than adults
b) CT scans are normal in approximately 20% of cases
c) Most foci demonstrated on MRI are clinically silent
d) Acute plaques of demyelination enhance for up to 8 weeks on MRI
e) In the spine, it has a predilection for the thoracic region

25 Regarding the leukodystrophies, which of the following are true?
a) Demyelination in adrenoleukodystrophy is usually first seen in the occipital lobes
b) Macrocephaly is typical of Canavan's disease
c) Metachromatic leukodystrophy is the most common inherited leukodystrophy
d) Classically, on CT, low-density basal ganglia are seen in Krabbe's disease
e) Enhancement following contrast administration is seen in Alexander's disease

26 Which of the following are true of intracranial aneurysms?
a) The incidence of saccular (berry) aneurysms is increased in aortic coarctation
b) Saccular aneurysms are multiple in approximately 50% of cases
c) Giant (larger than 2.5 cm) saccular aneurysms usually present following a subarachnoid haemorrhage (SAH)
d) Fusiform aneurysms typically affect the anterior circulation
e) Mycotic aneurysms are usually found in vessels distal to the circle of Willis

27 Which of the following are true of SAH?
a) No underlying cause can be identified in 5%–15% of cases
b) MRI is more sensitive than CT in the first 48 hours
c) Only 50% of all SAHs remain visible on CT scans performed 1 week after the event
d) SAH with an interhemispheric main clot suggests a bleed from an aneurysm of the anterior cerebral artery (ACA)
e) Repeated SAHs classically cause meninges that are hyperintense on T2-weighted imaging

28 Regarding intracranial vascular malformations, which of the following are true?
a) Arteriovenous malformations (AVMs) are multiple in 30% of cases
b) More than 70% of AVMs ultimately receive their blood supply from the internal cerebral artery
c) Capillary telangiectasia is most common in the pons and cerebellum
d) Cavernous haemangiomas have a characteristic low signal rim on T2-weighted imaging
e) Vein of Galen varices secondary to a thalamic AVM typically present in neonates

29 Concerning intracranial haematoma, which of the following are true?
a) An underlying skull fracture is detected in 85%–95% of epidural haematomata
b) An underlying skull fracture is detected in more than 30% of subdural haematomata
c) Hypertensive haemorrhage is most common in lobar white matter
d) Oxyhaemoglobin is isointense on T1-weighted imaging and hyperintense on T2-weighted imaging
e) Haemosiderin is hypointense on T1-weighted and T2-weighted imaging

30 Regarding head trauma, which of the following are true?
a) Diffuse axonal injury is most commonly seen at lobar grey–white matter junctions
b) Cerebral contusions are multiple in 70% of cases
c) Posttraumatic diffuse cerebral oedema is more common in adults than children
d) Posttraumatic extracranial ICA dissections commonly involve the bulb region
e) Traumatic SAH is typically less extensive than when secondary to an aneurysm

31 Which of the following statements about nonglial tumours are true?
- a) Dysembryoplastic neuroepithelial tumours are most common in white matter
- b) Gangliogliomas undergo cystic change in 30%–50% of cases
- c) A pineal germinoma is usually slightly hypodense on unenhanced CT
- d) A pineoblastoma typically contains a central foci of fat
- e) Primitive neuroectodermal tumours (PNET) usually enhance avidly on CT

32 Which of the following are more typical of thyroid eye disease than orbital pseudotumour?
- a) Bilateral disease
- b) Involvement of the muscular tendons
- c) The presence of proptosis
- d) Enlargement of the lacrimal gland
- e) A marked response to steroids

33 Within the orbit, which of the following are true?
- a) Orbital melanoma is classically hyperintense on T1-weighted and T2-weighted MRI
- b) Norrie's disease is associated with persistent hyperplastic primary vitreous (PHPV)
- c) Coats' disease typically presents in males aged 6–8 years
- d) About 80% of optic nerve gliomas occur in the first decade of life
- e) About 90% of capillary haemangiomas are associated with a skin angioma

34 Which of the following are true of retinoblastoma?
- a) Approximately one third of cases are hereditary
- b) The nonhereditary type usually presents before the age of 5 years
- c) Calcification is seen in less than 50% of cases
- d) The optic nerve is involved in 25% of cases
- e) On MRI, the tumour is distinctly hypointense on T2-weighted imaging

35 Concerning infections of the spine, which of the following are true?
- a) *Staphylococcus aureus* is the most common cause of infectious spondylitis
- b) Pyogenic spondylitis is most common in the thoracic spine
- c) In pyogenic spondylitis the intervertebral disc is typically high signal on T2-weighted imaging
- d) Paraspinal soft-tissue changes are characteristically minimal in tuberculous spondylitis
- e) *Brucella* spondylitis has a predilection for the cervical spine

36 Regarding spinal tumours, which of the following are true?
- a) Approximately 50% of chordomas are located in the sacrum
- b) Ependymomas are typically hypointense to the spinal cord on T1-weighted imaging
- c) Spinal astrocytomas are most commonly located in the cervicothoracic region
- d) Spinal meningiomas calcify less frequently than intracranial meningiomas
- e) Most vertebral body haemangiomas give a high signal on T1- and T2-weighted imaging

37 Which of the following are true of diastematomyelia?
a) The two hemicords share a thecal sac in approximately 50% of cases
b) An osseous spur is seen on CT in more than 80% of cases
c) There is no association with the Chiari II malformation
d) The cleft is located below T9 in 85% of cases
e) In 75% of cases, the conus medullaris lies below L2

38 Posterior vertebral scalloping occurs in which of the following?
a) Ankylosing spondylitis
b) Hurler's syndrome
c) Down's syndrome
d) Achondroplasia
e) Hypothyroidism

39 Which of the following are classical associations?
a) Coronal cleft vertebral bodies and chondrodysplasia punctata
b) Central anterior vertebral body beaks and Hurler's syndrome
c) Diffuse platyspondyly and osteogenesis imperfecta
d) A solitary ivory vertebral body and Hodgkin's disease
e) Klippel–Feil syndrome and deafness

40 Which of the following statements are true regarding trauma to the spinal cord?
a) Cord damage is unusual in the Jefferson (vertical compression) fracture of the axis
b) The flexion teardrop fracture is a stable injury
c) Chance fractures are most common at L2 and L3
d) In acute trauma to the spinal cord, areas of hypointensity on T2-weighted imaging imply a poor prognosis
e) Nerve root avulsions are most common in the thoracic spine

Answers

1 a) **False** The corpus callosum develops from front to back (anterior to posterior), except for the rostrum, which develops last. Therefore, isolated agenesis of the anteriorly positioned genu, unlike the rostrum or splenium, is very rare.

   b) **True** Hence, the bones of the skull vault are involved in cleidocranial dysostosis, but are spared in achondroplasia.

   c) **True** The conus is located at L4/5 at 16 weeks gestational age and at L1/2 at more than 3 months of age. Location of the conus at or below L3 in an adult is suggestive of a tethered cord.

   d) **True** This is felt to be secondary to neurosecretory vesicles, which pass down to the posterior pituitary from the hypothalamus. The posterior lobe of the pituitary is isointense on T1-weighted imaging in 10% of cases. An absent T1 high signal is associated with central diabetes insipidus and compressive anterior pituitary lesions.

   e) **True** CSP is a midline CSF cavity within the septum pellucidum. It is present in 80% of term infants. Rarely, it may enlarge and cause hydrocephalus. In the absence of a CSP a septum pellucidum larger than 3 mm is suggestive of an infiltrating neoplasm. Cavum vergae is a posterior extension of CSP and is seen in 30% of term infants.

2 a) **True** The biparietal diameter is measured from the outer edge of the near-field calvarial table to the inner edge of the far-field calvarial table. It is used from 12 weeks gestational age, but is less reliable in the third trimester.

   b) **True** The cisterna magna normally measures 3–10 mm deep. If seen, it almost completely excludes underlying spina bifida. It can be obliterated in Arnold–Chiari malformation when the cerebellum wraps around the posterior brain stem (the 'banana sign').

   c) **True** Much earlier diagnosis is difficult, as the normal skull does not ossify until about 14 weeks gestational age. Ultrasound shows symmetrical absence of the bony calvarium, a cranial soft tissue mass, bulging frog-like eyes and polyhydramnios in about 50% of cases.

   d) **False** They are seen in up to 4% of antenatal ultrasound scans (50% at autopsy). They frequently resolve spontaneously, but can be associated with trisomy 18 and 21, triploidy and Klinefelter's syndrome.

   e) **False** Acutely it is echogenic, but after 2–3 weeks the echogenicity decreases (starting centrally). It may completely resolve or leave a residual cyst. More than 90% of germinal matrix bleeds occur by the sixth day of life (35% on day 1). The most common site of germinal matrix haemorrhage is around the caudothalamic notch. Ultrasound sensitivity is more than 90% for larger than 5 mm bleeds and less than 30% if the bleed is smaller than 5 mm.

3 a) **False** It is lined by heterotopic grey matter, indicating that the cleft forms before the end of the period of neuronal migration (compare this with acquired porencephaly), which for the cerebral cortex lasts 8–16 weeks gestational age.

   b) **True** Less commonly, the corpus callosum is absent.

   c) **True** It is also seen in Miller–Dieker and Norman–Roberts syndromes.

   d) **True** Nodular heterotopias are unlike the subependymal nodules seen in tuberous sclerosis, which can enhance or calcify and are not always precisely isointense to grey matter.

   e) **True** Localised changes are more common than generalised changes and often involve arterial territories, especially the middle cerebral artery.

4 a) **False** This abnormality results in hydranencephaly, in which there is no anterior cerebral mantle or facial anomaly and the falx cerebri and thalami are normal.

   b) **True**

   c) **False**

   d) **False**

   e) **True**

   b–e) Holoprosencephaly results from partial/complete lack of cleavage of the developing forebrain and is divided into three types: alobar, semilobar and lobar. The alobar type is most severe and is characterised by fused cerebral hemispheres with an anterior cup-shaped brain, a single monoventricle, fused thalami and absent corpus callosum, fornix, optic tracts and olfactory bulbs (the midbrain, brain stem and cerebellum are normal). The semilobar type is of intermediate severity and is characterised by partial cleavage into hemispheres, monoventricles with rudimentary occipital and temporal horns. The falx cerebri may be present posteriorly and the thalami are variably fused. The lobar type is the least severe and is characterised by lateral ventricles that are almost normal, but frontal horns point inferiorly and may be 'squared'. The septum pellucidum is absent in all three subtypes. The incidence is equal in males and females and is associated with: chromosome abnormalities (trisomy 13 and 18 are most common), polyhydramnios (60%), and renal and cardiac anomalies. Facial anomalies are also common, ranging from cyclopia to hypotelorism, and they usually correlate with the severity of the brain abnormality. Septo-optic dysplasia (absence of the septum pellucidum and hypoplastic anterior optic pathways) may be considered a mild form of lobar holoprosencephaly.

5 a) **False** Cystic dilatation and posterior extension of the fourth ventricle lead to an enlarged posterior fossa with a high tentorium, straight sinus and torcular herophili. In the Dandy–Walker variant, the posterior fossa is normal size.

   b) **True** The fourth ventricle opens dorsally between the separated and hypoplastic cerebellar hemispheres. The pons may be hypoplastic or anteriorly displaced.

   c) **False** The vermian remnant is superiorly displaced. There is an association with hypoplasia and aplasia (total in 25% and partial in 75%) of the cerebellar vermis.

   d) **True** An associated CNS abnormality is seen in 70% of cases of Dandy–Walker malformation: callosal dysgenesis (20%–25%), holoprosencephaly (25%), grey matter heterotopias or syringomyelia.

   e) **True** Other non-CNS associations include Klippel–Feil syndrome, Cornelia de Lange syndrome, cleft palate and cardiac anomalies.

6 a) **False** The Chiari I malformation is characterised by displacement of the cerebellar tonsils below the foramen magnum (more than 5 mm). The Chiari II malformation is associated with myelomeningocele in more than 95% of cases.

b) **False** The Chiari II malformation is characterised by a small posterior fossa with a caudally displaced brain stem, which results in a small fourth ventricle that is vertically elongated with a narrowed antero–posterior diameter.

c) **False** The foramen magnum is enlarged, as is the upper spinal canal in 75% of cases.

d) **True** Lacunar skull (lückenschädel) occurs in 85% of cases, is most prominent at birth and near the torcular herophili and largely disappears by 6 months of age.

e) **True** The rare Chiari III type is the association of a low occipital/high cervical encephalocoele with a Chiari II malformation. Death in infancy is usual.

7 a) **False**
b) **True**
c) **False**
d) **False**
e) **True**

This sporadically occurring phakomatosis is characterised by capillary venous angiomas involving the face and the ipsilateral eye, and leptomeninges. Other features include: seizures, mental retardation, ipsilateral glaucoma, choroidal haemangiomata, buphthalmos, contralateral hemiparesis and, rarely, angiomatous malformations of the intestines, kidneys, spleen, ovaries and lungs. The intracranial lesions are most common in the parietal–occipital lobes, occasionally the frontal lobes, and, rarely, the posterior fossa. Cortical calcification is unusual before the age of 2 years. Ipsilateral choroid plexus enlargement, vault thickening, and prominence of the paranasal sinuses and mastoid air cells can be seen.

8 a) **False** About 50% of cases are inherited in an autosomal dominant manner secondary to a deletion from the long arm of chromosome 22 (50% are spontaneous mutations). Chromosome 17 defects can lead to NF-1.

b) **True** It can also be diagnosed if there is a first-degree relative with NF-2, plus either a single acoustic schwannoma or any two of schwannoma, glioma, neurofibroma, meningioma, or juvenile posterior subcapsular lens opacity. NF-2 causes lesions of Schwann cells and meninges (e.g. schwannomas and meningiomas), whereas NF-1 causes lesions of neurons and astrocytes.

c) **True** Isolated schwannomas can occur in other cranial nerves, except for optic and olfactory nerves, which are really brain tracts and lack Schwann cells.

d) **False** In NF-1, but not NF-2, optic nerve gliomas are seen in 5%–15% of patients.

e) **True** Conversely, in NF-1, an intramedullary lesion is more likely to be a low-grade astrocytoma. Other NF-1 spinal lesions include neurofibromas and lateral meningoceles secondary to dural ectasia.

9 a) **False**
b) **False**
c) **True**
d) **False**
e) **False**

Four major types of intracranial lesion are recognised.
- Cortical tubers are detected on MRI in 95% of patients; 5% enhance and they are not premalignant. MRI characteristics change with age, but in older children and adults they are isointense to brain parenchyma on T1-weighted imaging, and hyperintense to brain parenchyma on T2-weighted imaging.
- White matter abnormalities are disorganised, dysplastic heterotopic lesions that enhance in less than 20% of cases, and which have a similar MRI signal to cortical tubers.
- Subependymal nodules are found in 95% of cases, most commonly along the third ventricle near the caudate nucleus, and rarely in the third or fourth ventricles. They increase in number and degree of calcification with time.
- Giant cell astrocytomas occur in 15% of cases, are almost always located around the foramen of Munro, are frequently calcified and enhance avidly but heterogeneously. They enlarge with time and often cause hydrocephalus.

10 All false Colloid cysts account for about 1% of intracranial tumours, have an approximately equal gender incidence, and are present in young adults (aged 20–40 years) but rare in children. They present with positional headaches, gait apraxia and changes in mental status. They are thought to be of neuro-ectodermal origin and arise almost exclusively from the anterior portion of the third ventricle, inferior to the septum pellucidum and between the foramina of Munro (hence the predisposition to hydrocephalus). They contain mucoproteinaceous material, and are hyperdense on CT in two thirds of cases and isodense in the remaining third. The MRI characteristics vary, but the most common appearance is T1-weighted hyperintensity and T2-weighted hypointensity. Enhancement is rare, although it has been described peripherally.

11 a) **False** Glioblastoma multiforme are benign lesions that result from duplication/splitting of the arachnoid membrane (congenital or postsurgery, posthaemorrhage or postinfection). They are most common in the middle cranial fossa (about 60%), while 5%–10% of cases occur in the posterior fossa.

b) **True** Lesions typically occur off midline; 40%–50% are found in the CPA (they are the third most common CPA mass after acoustic schwannomas and meningiomas) and 5%–10% occur in the middle cranial fossa.

c) **True** Arachnoid cysts are isointense/isodense to CSF (unless haemorrhage occurs). Epidermoid cysts are generally isointense to CSF, but can be hyperintense on proton density-weighted MRI.

d) **True** Conversely, arachnoid cysts typically displace, but do not encase, structures.

e) **True** 10%–25% of epidermoid cysts calcify and occasional peripheral enhancement is described. Arachnoid cysts do not enhance or calcify.

12 a) **True**   It accounts for 50% of all astrocytomas and 1%–2% of all malignancies.
   b) **False**   It occurs at all ages, but the peak incidence is at age 65–75 years. It is more common in Caucasians.
   c) **True**   It is also associated with Turcot syndrome and Li–Fraumeni syndrome.
   d) **False**   It is most commonly located in the white matter of the cerebral hemispheres, particularly fronto-temporal.
   e) **False**   Peritumoural oedema is usually striking. The signal intensity and density of the tumour itself are typically very heterogeneous.

13 a) **False**   Macroadenomas are defined as those more than 10 mm in diameter, but they frequently present because of mass effect. They are commonly hormonally inactive.
   b) **False**   ACTH-secreting tumours account for about 15% of microadenomas, as do growth hormone (GH)-secreting tumours. The most common type of pituitary adenoma is a prolactinoma (30%), followed by null-cell type (25%).
   c) **True**   This is unlike craniopharyngiomas, which calcify in up to 90% of cases.
   d) **False**   About 65%–90% are hypodense/hypointense to the normal pituitary on early postcontrast images. Macroadenomas usually enhance well, but mixed density/intensity lesions can be seen after haemorrhage or cyst formation.
   e) **True**   The so-called malignant adenomas represent less than 1% of all pituitary adenomas. The most common malignant pituitary tumour is a metastasis.

14 a) **False**   More than 50% present in childhood/adolescence, with a peak incidence at 8–12 years of age and a second smaller peak in middle age. Headache and growth delay are the most common presentations. It has an equal gender incidence.
   b) **False**   They are benign tumours from the epithelial remnants along Rathke's pouch.
   c) **True**   They are suprasellar in 20% of cases and suprasellar/sellar in 70% of cases. Occasionally, they are ectopically located in the floor of the third ventricle (more common in adults) and in the sphenoid bone.
   d) **False**   On CT, calcification is seen in 90% of children and 50% of adults. In 90% of cases, they are predominantly cystic masses with nodular/rim enhancement.
   e) **True**   They are characterised by heterogeneously enhancing lesions with a variable T1-weighted signal depending on the cyst content (protein, blood, cholesterol), but are usually hypointense.

15 a) **True** They are three times more common in women than men. They can enlarge in pregnancy and are associated with breast carcinoma, factors that suggest they are sex hormone-dependent. Radiation therapy is also a risk factor.

b) **True** Typical locations include the cerebral hemispheres (25%), parafalcine (20%), sphenoid ridge (20%), spine (12%), frontobasal (10%) and posterior fossa (10%). Less common locations include the CPA, the optic nerve sheath (adult females), the ventricular system (lateral > third > fourth), and rarely extradural (e.g. paranasal sinuses, mediastinum). They are multifocal in up to 10% of cases.

c) **False** They are hyperdense (75% of cases) or isodense (25% of cases) on unenhanced CT and avid enhancement is seen in 90%. Surrounding oedema is seen in 60% of cases, calcification in about 20%, and cystic areas in 15%.

d) **False** There is an almost 100% detection rate with gadolinium-enhanced MRI. The signal varies, but is typically hypointense or isointense on T1-weighted imaging and isointense or hyperintense on T2-weighted imaging. A dural tail is suggestive of, but not pathognomonic for, intracranial meningiomas and is seen in 60% of cases.

e) **False** About 1%–2% are frankly malignant. No clear radiological signs predict malignancy, although T2-weighted hyperintense tumours tend to be more atypical.

16 a) **True** They are also associated with ataxia telangiectasia.

b) **True** It accounts for 30% of posterior fossa tumours in children, with a smaller peak in the third decade of life. There is a slight male predominance (M:F = 2:1).

c) **False** They are typically located in the cerebellar vermis (75%) and cerebellar hemispheres (25%). The lateral cerebellar location is more common in the older age group.

d) **False** This is more typical of haemangioblastoma than medulloblastoma. The 'typical' CT appearance of medulloblastoma is seen in only 50% of cases: hyperdense precontrast with strong enhancement. Atypical features (more likely in the older age group) include cystic change (15%), calcification (10%) and nonenhancement (3%). The MRI signal is variable; it is usually hypointense on T1-weighted imaging and hypointense to hyperintense on T2-weighted imaging.

e) **False** Disseminated disease is seen in 50% of cases. Common metastatic sites include the brain or spine via CSF seeding, but also distant sites, including primarily the bone (lytic/sclerotic lesions).

17 a) **False** Although patients typically present with sensorineural hearing loss, the tumour arises from the vestibular component in 85% of cases and the cochlear in 15%.

b) **False** They are diagnostic of NF-2, which is also present in up to 25% of patients with unilateral lesions.

c) **True** This is unlike classically hyperdense or isodense meningioma, and hypodense epidermoid.

d) **True** CPA meningiomas also enhance avidly, but 50% are isointense on T2-weighted imaging.

e) **False** Calcification is rare (unlike meningioma), but cystic change is seen in 15% of cases.

18 a) **False**   Metastases normally account for up to 35% of intracranial tumours.
   b) **True**   Other locations include the subarachnoid space (15%), skull (5%) and dura (rare).
   c) **False**   Between 60% and 85% of metastatic lesions are multiple.
   d) **True**   The most common primary sites of intracranial metastases are lung, breast, colorectal, kidney and melanoma.
   e) **False**   A paraneoplastic syndrome (seen in 2%–3% of patients with small cell lung cancer) is the most common cause of limbic encephalitis. The CT is usually normal. A high signal on T2-weighted imaging may be seen in the medial temporal lobes.

19 All true   Other causes include:
   - idiopathic/senescent (most common)
   - metabolic (e.g. hyperparathyroidism, pseudo- and pseudopseudohypoparathyroidism)
   - infection (e.g. TORCH syndrome [toxoplasmosis, other infections, rubella, cytomegalovirus and herpes simplex], tuberculosis, cysticercosis)
   - toxic (e.g. lead, carbon monoxide, chemotherapy, radiotherapy)
   - postanoxic (e.g. birth anoxia, cardiac arrest)
   - miscellaneous (e.g. systemic lupus erythematosus, tuberous sclerosis, mitochondrial disease, Down's syndrome)

20 a) **True**   The caudate nucleus, claustrum and amygdaloid body are the other constituents of the basal ganglia. The major blood supply is via the lenticulostriate and thalamoperforating arteries.
   b) **False**   The basal ganglia are low in density, as the copper deposition leads to spongy degeneration and cavitation. They are high signal on T2-weighted imaging. Other causes of high signal on T2-weighted imaging of basal ganglia include: lymphoma, hypoxia, venous infarction, Huntington's chorea (also causes caudate atrophy), Hallervorden–Spatz disease, mitochondrial diseases, aminoacidopathies and toxins (e.g. methanol, carbon monoxide, hydrogen sulphide).
   c) **True**   Low attenuation basal ganglia can also be seen in poisoning (carbon monoxide, methanol, cyanide, hydrogen sulphide), hypoxia, hypotension (lacunar infarcts) and Wilson's disease.
   d) **True**   They are also seen with dystrophic calcification, liver failure and total parenteral nutrition (manganese).
   e) **True**   They can also occur in old age, Parkinson's disease and following childhood hypoxia.

21 a) **False**   The most common CNS manifestation is meningitis. Tuberculomas occur in 25% of cases (solitary lesions in more than 70%). Vasculitis and infarction may also be seen. CNS involvement is usually secondary to haematogenous spread from the lungs.

   b) **True**   Cortical/subcortical location of tuberculomas is typical. In children, cerebellar lesions are common.

   c) **True**   In patients with sarcoidosis, CNS involvement occurs in 1%–8% clinically and about 15% at autopsy. Sarcoidosis affects the meninges and cranial nerves to a greater extent than the brain parenchyma. The pituitary gland, optic chiasm and hypothalamus are also commonly involved.

   d) **True**   Granulomatous meningitis is also seen in tuberculosis, sarcoidosis and many fungal causes of meningitis, such as candidiasis, blastomycosis, actinomycosis, nocardiosis, aspergillosis and cryptococcosis. Meninges appear thickened and are hyperintense on T2-weighted imaging. It may be associated with hydrocephalus, cerebritis and abscesses.

   e) **True**   Granulomatous angiitis is an uncommon vasculitis of unknown aetiology. An association with CNS infections and tumours has been reported. Imaging findings are nonspecific.

22 a) **True**   The mortality rate is 50%–70%, with significant morbidity in survivors.

   b) **True**   In neonates, HSV-2 is acquired during parturition or transplacentally and manifests several weeks after birth as nonfocal encephalitis. HSV-1 affects children and adults, and is commonly secondary to reactivation of latent virus in the trigeminal ganglion. Infection is usually focal and involves the limbic system.

   c) **False**   Adult HSE is often initially unilateral, but is typically followed by less severe contralateral disease (sequential bilaterality).

   d) **True**   On MRI, the signal abnormalities (hyperintensity on T2-weighted imaging in the temporal lobe/cingulate gyrus) often extend into the insular cortex, but spare the putamen.

   e) **False**   Peripheral/gyral/cisternal enhancement may persist for several months.

23 a) **False**   HIVE is caused by HIV infection itself and is seen in up to 60% of AIDS cases.

   b) **True**   Atrophy is the most common finding. HIVE usually affects deep white matter and spares grey matter. Lesions are typically multifocal, bilateral, asymmetrical, nonenhancing, CT hypodense and hyperintense on T2-weighted imaging with no mass effect.

   c) **False**   PML is caused by papovavirus (principally the JC virus) and preferentially involves subcortical white matter (usually parietal and occipital) before spreading centrally. Grey matter is involved in up to 50% of cases. Lesions typically do not enhance or exert a mass effect. Death usually occurs within 6 months.

   d) **True**   Toxoplasmosis is the most common opportunistic CNS infection in AIDS patients. Lesions classically enhance and affect the basal ganglia and cerebral hemispheres near the corticomedullary junction. Features favouring lymphoma over toxoplasmosis include a periventricular location and subependymal spread.

   e) **False**   This fungal infection occurs in 2%–5% of patients with AIDS, and the meninges, basal ganglia and midbrain are most frequently involved.

24 a) **True** Only 10% of plaques are infratentorial in adults, whereas 85% of adults demonstrate periventricular lesions, which are classically oriented perpendicular to the long axis of the brain and lateral ventricles (Dawson's fingers).

   b) **True** On CT, nonspecific atrophy is seen in 45% of cases. Plaques are hypodense or isodense and acutely show transient enhancement for about 2 weeks.

   c) **True** This reflects the high sensitivity of MRI (approximately 85%).

   d) **True** This reflects the breakdown in the blood–brain barrier. Enhancement is usually solid or ring-like and may mimic a tumour or abscess. Chronic plaques do not enhance due to restoration of the blood–brain barrier.

   e) **False** The cervical spine is affected in up to 50% of cases and in 12% of those without intracranial disease.

25 a) **True** A defect of fatty acid oxidation leads to a build up of long-chain fatty acids. Adrenoleukodystrophy is more common in males than females, and typically occurs age 3–10 years. The most common mode of inheritance is X-linked recessive. The disease starts around the lateral trigones.

   b) **True** Macrocephaly is also seen in Alexander's disease.

   c) **True** Metachromatic leukodystrophy is seen in 1:100 000 neonates. It is autosomal recessive and is caused by a deficiency of arylsulphatase A. In 70% of cases, it is present at 1–2 years. Death occurs 1–4 years later. It involves the periventricular white matter and cerebellum, but spares the subcortical white matter.

   d) **False** Basal ganglia usually have increased density. Symmetrical high-density foci can also be seen in the corona radiata and cerebellum, and the white matter can be of decreased density.

   e) **True** Enhancement is also seen in adrenoleukodystrophy.

26 a) **True** An increased incidence is also seen in the presence of anomalous cranial vessels, as well as in Marfan's syndrome, Ehlers–Danlos syndrome, autosomal dominant polycystic kidney disease and fibromuscular dysplasia.

   b) **False** About 15%–20% of cases of berry aneurysms are multiple. A strong female predominance exists with multiple aneurysms (overall F:M = 5:1, but for more than 3 aneurysms F:M = 11:1).

   c) **False** They tend to present with symptoms related to their mass effect.

   d) **False** Fusiform aneurysms more usually affect the vertebrobasilar system and are secondary to atherosclerosis.

   e) **True** About 65% occur distal to the circle of Willis. Causes include subacute bacterial endocarditis and intravenous drug abuse (65%), acute bacterial endocarditis (10%), septic thrombophlebitis (10%) and meningitis (10%). They are more common in children than adults and are multiple in 20% of cases.

27 a) **True**   These cases are rarely recurrent and have a good prognosis. Other causes include: ruptured berry aneurysm (75%), AVM (10%), hypertension (5%), trauma, anticoagulation, tumour, spinal AVM and intracranial infection.

    b) **False**   The converse is true, as deoxyhaemoglobin is almost isointense to normal brain. CT is 60%–95% accurate in the first 4–5 days. MRI is more accurate than CT for chronic SAH.

    c) **True**   This is because 90% of extravasated blood is cleared from the CSF within 1 week. Consider rebleeding if SAH remains visible after 2 weeks.

    d) **True**   Other clues as to the original source of the haemorrhage include sylvian fissure blood and middle cerebral artery (MCA) aneurysm(s), blood in the fourth ventricle and ruptured posterior fossa aneurysm(s).

    e) **False**   Haemosiderin deposition on the meninges leads to leptomeningeal siderosis, which is hypointense on T2-weighted imaging. This can lead to neurological dysfunction.

28 a) **False**   In fact, 98% are solitary. AVMs are characterised by an abnormal network of arteries and veins with no intervening capillary bed. Peak incidence occurs between ages 20 and 40 years. About 90% are supratentorial.

    b) **True**   Approximately 25% receive their blood supply from the dural branches of the external cerebral artery.

    c) **True**   Abnormal dilated capillaries are separated by normal brain tissue. Multiple lesions are the rule. They are associated with Osler–Weber–Rendu syndrome. CT is often normal. MRI shows multiple T2-hypointense foci if haemorrhage has occurred.

    d) **True**   This is due to a rim of haemosiderin. Combined with a mixed signal intensity core, secondary to blood products of varying age, the lesion has a characteristic 'popcorn' appearance. About 80% are supratentorial and 50%–80% are multiple.

    e) **False**   AVM-type varices typically present in older infants with developmental delay or haemorrhage. Vein of Galen malformations are a complex group of vascular anomalies characterised by dilatation of the vein of Galen, either due to a direct fistula or distant AVM. Fistula types tend to present neonatally with congestive heart failure.

29 a) **True** The temporo-parietal location is most common (75%). About 90% are secondary to a tear of the middle meningeal artery and the rest result from a tear of the meningeal vein or sinus. They do not cross suture lines, but may cross dural reflections. The mortality rate is 5%.

b) **False** Associated fractures are rarely seen (less than 10%). They result from tearing of bridging veins of the subdural space. They cross suture lines, but not dural reflections. They are bilateral in 20% of adults and 80% of children. The mortality rate is 30%–90%.

c) **False** Hypertensive haemorrhage is seen in men aged 60–80 years. Common locations include the basal ganglia (60%–80%), thalamus (10%–20%), pons (5%–10%), dentate nuclei (1%–5%) and hemispheres (1%–2%). It involves the penetrating arteries off the MCA. The mortality rate is 50%.

d) **True** Oxyhaemoglobin (present up to 12 hours following the event) is diamagnetic. Its appearance reflects the water in blood. At this stage, detection by MRI is less sensitive than CT.

e) **True** Haemosiderin forms about 2 weeks after the event (starts at the margins of the haematoma) and may remain permanently. Methaemoglobin forms 3–14 days after the event and is hyperintense on T1-weighted imaging.

30 a) **True** It also occurs in the splenium of the corpus callosum and dorsolateral brainstem. It is seen in severe head trauma where rotational shearing forces lead to axonal disruption. Initial CTs are normal in 50%–85% of cases. MRI shows a multifocal high signal on T2-weighted imaging.

b) **False** They are multiple in 30% of cases. They involve the frontal and temporal lobes. MRI is more sensitive than CT and shows hypodense areas with dense foci due to petechial haemorrhage.

c) **False** Posttraumatic diffuse cerebral oedema is seen in 10%–20% of severe brain injuries and is nearly twice as common in children as adults. It usually develops after 24–48 hours and has a mortality rate of 50%.

d) **False** Posttraumatic extracranial ICA dissections usually spare the bulb and arise 2 cm distal to the common carotid bifurcation.

e) **True** Traumatic SAH rarely induces vasospasm. It may arise from an extension of brain contusions.

31 a) **False** These are rare, benign tumours that affect children and frequently cause epilepsy. They are cortically based (commonly in the temporal lobe) and are associated with cortical dysplasia. They exert little mass effect and do not enhance. They give a low signal on T1-weighted imaging and a high signal on T2-weighted imaging.

b) **True** Gangliogliomas are benign and 80% occur under the age of 30 years. They are most common in the cerebral hemispheres: temporal > frontal > parietal. About 30% calcify. They may cause pressure erosion of the overlying vault.

c) **False** A pineal germinoma is usually slightly hyperdense on precontrast CT. They enhance on CT and MRI. Incidence is much greater in males than females. They usually present in patients between 10 and 30 years of age. They account for about 33% of all pineal region neoplasms and nearly 80% of pineal germ-cell tumours. Other pineal region tumours of germ cell origin include: teratoma (20% of pineal germ-cell tumours), choriocarcinoma (4%) and embryonal cell tumours (4%). Apart from germ-cell tumours, the other main category of pineal region neoplasms is pineal cell tumours, such as pineocytoma (benign) and pineoblastoma (very malignant).

d) **False** Fat is typical of pineal teratomas. Pineoblastomas may contain some peripherally displaced normal pineal calcification ('exploded' pattern).

e) **True** PNET tumours (e.g. pineoblastoma, medulloblastoma, ependymoblastoma and retinoblastoma) are aggressive, enhancing and undifferentiated lesions that are common in children and frequently metastasise via the CSF.

32 a) **True** Thyroid eye disease is bilateral in 85% of cases, whereas pseudotumour is bilateral in 15%.

b) **False** Unlike orbital pseudotumour, thyroid eye disease typically spares the muscular tendons. The order of involvement is inferior rectus > medial > superior > lateral. The involved muscles give a high signal on T2-weighted imaging.

c) **False** Proptosis occurs in both conditions. It is painful in pseudotumour. It is defined as a globe protrusion larger than 21 mm anterior to the interzygomatic line at the level of the lens.

d) **False** The lacrimal gland is involved in 5% of cases of pseudotumour.

e) **False** Although both conditions may respond to steroids, orbital pseudotumour usually shows a dramatic response. In thyroid eye disease, spontaneous resolution is seen in up to 90% of cases; 10% develop corneal ulceration/optic neuropathy.

33 a) **False**   Orbital melanoma is classically T1 hyperintense (because of melanin) but T2 hypointense on MRI. It is hyperdense on CT, enhances moderately and retinal detachments are common.

   b) **True**   This rare, X-linked, recessive disease is also associated with seizures, a low IQ and deafness. CT shows microphthalmia, hyperdense vitreous and a central structure in the vitreous (a remnant of the hyaloid artery). Unlike retinoblastoma, there is no calcification and PHPV tends to be hyperintense on T2-weighted imaging.

   c) **True**   Coats' disease is a congenital vascular malformation leading to retinal telangiectasia and detachment. The incidence in males is twice that in females. It is unilateral in 90% of cases. There is no focal mass or calcification.

   d) **True**   Peak incidence is at age 5 years. Optic nerve gliomas are well-differentiated pilocytic astrocytomas. They occur in 15% of patients with NF-1 – often bilaterally. They enhance and calcify much less than optic nerve meningiomas, which predominantly affect females (80% of cases), peak in incidence in the fourth decade and are associated with NF-2.

   e) **True**   Capillary haemangiomas account for 10%–15% of paediatric orbital tumours. They grow for less than 1 year and then involute and enhance. The superior nasal quadrant is the most common location.

34 a) **True**   Such cases are secondary to defects (monosomy/deletions) in chromosome 13. Hereditary cases present earlier and are more likely to be bilateral (70% of cases) than nonhereditary cases (30%). The trilateral type is bilateral disease plus pineoblastoma.

   b) **True**   About 70% of nonhereditary cases present before 3 years and 98% before 5 years (mean: 18 months). The incidence is equal in males and females.

   c) **False**   Calcification is seen in 50%–95% of cases and its presence is a favourable prognostic sign. Contrast enhancement is a poor prognostic sign.

   d) **True**   Mortality is less than 10% if the optic nerve is spared, but 50% if it is significantly involved.

   e) **True**   The tumour is isointense or mildly hyperintense on T1-weighted imaging relative to the vitreous.

35 a) **True**   *S. aureus* accounts for 60% of cases of pyogenic infection. Other causes include *Enterobacter* organisms (30%), *Escherichia coli*, *Pseudomonas* and *Klebsiella*. Most instances arise from haematogenous spread. Infection in adults starts in the end plates, whereas in children it starts in the disc.

    b) **False**   Pyogenic spondylitis can occur anywhere in the spine, but most commonly affects the lumbar spine. The sacrum and cervical spine are less commonly involved. It affects multiple levels in 25% of cases.

    c) **True**   T1-weighted imaging shows a narrowed disc with a low signal in the adjacent vertebral body.

    d) **False**   The converse is true. Up to 80% of cases (as opposed to 20% in pyogenic infections) involve a large paraspinal abscess, which is often calcified. The lower thoracic and upper lumbar spine areas are the most frequently involved sites. Paraspinal soft tissue changes are more indolent than pyogenic infections and reactive bony sclerosis is a late feature. Discs may be spared and skip lesions are common.

    e) **False**   The lumbar spine (especially L4) is the most common site of *Brucella* spondylitis (70% of cases). It is difficult to distinguish from tuberculous spondylitis, but features in favour of brucellosis include lower lumbar region-only involvement, normal paraspinal soft tissues and absent gibbus.

36 a) **True**   Chordomas are rare, slow-growing and locally aggressive enhancing tumours, which arise from notochordal remnants. A total of 35% occur in the clivus and 15% in the spine (particularly cervical and thoracic). Tumours have a large soft-tissue component and calcification occurs in 30%–70% of cases.

    b) **True**   Ependymomas are the most common primary spinal tumour, accounting for about 66% of all intramedullary tumours. They are usually located around the lower cord, conus and filum terminale. The incidence is greater in females. The incidence peaks between 40 and 60 years of age. They are associated with NF-2, are slow-growing, and produce bony scalloping in 30% of cases. Tumours enhance and are partially cystic in 50% of cases, and evidence of prior haemorrhage is seen in 65% of cases on MRI.

    c) **True**   Spinal astrocytomas are the second most common primary spinal tumour, accounting for about 30% of all intramedullary tumours. The incidence is greater in males than females, and peaks between 20 and 30 years of age. They are associated with NF-1, bony remodelling occurs in 50% of cases, and cystic regions are found in 25%–35% of cases.

    d) **True**   Most spinal meningiomas occur in the thoracic spine (80%), in females (80%), and in patients aged over 40 years. About 10% cause bone erosion and 85% are intradural. Multiple tumours are associated with NF-2. Tumours are isointense to the spinal cord on T1- and T2-weighted imaging, and enhance avidly.

    e) **True**   Vertebral body haemangiomas occur in about 10% of the general population. The incidence is greater in females than males, and 70% of haemangiomas are solitary. They most commonly occur in the thoracic and lumbar spine, and may cause symptoms if they are very large. They are partly lytic, with a thick trabeculae 'corduroy' pattern on plain film and 'polka-dot' appearance on CT.

37 a) **True** This condition is characterised by sagittal clefting of the spinal cord or filum terminale into two hemicords, each of which contains a central canal, but only one dorsal and one ventral horn (compare with diplomyelia – true spinal cord duplication). The cord is usually single above and below the split.

b) **False** An osseous spur is seen on CT in only 50% of cases. In a smaller proportion of cases the spur is fibrous. The spur may traverse part of or the entire canal and may not be midline.

c) **False** Diastematomyelia occurs in 15%–20% of patients with Chiari II malformation. Other associations include myelomeningocele, hydromyelia, scoliosis, clubfoot, and cutaneous stigmata overlying the spine. Osseous abnormalities (hemi or block vertebra, narrow discs) are seen in more than 85% of cases.

d) **True** A cervical or upper thoracic location is rare.

e) **True** A tethered cord is seen in more than 50% of cases.

38 a) **True**
b) **True**
c) **False**
d) **True**
e) **False**

Posterior vertebral scalloping occurs secondary to:
- long-standing increased intraspinal pressure: tumours in the spinal canal, communicating hydrocephalus, syringomyelia
- mesenchymal tissue laxity and dural ectasia
- NF (local scalloping can also result from a neurofibroma), Marfan's syndrome, Ehlers–Danlos syndrome
- bone softening
- mucopolysaccharidoses (e.g. Hurler's syndrome, Morquio's syndrome and Sanfilippo's syndrome), acromegaly, achondroplasia, ankylosing spondylitis and osteogenesis imperfecta

39 a) **True** Coronal cleft vertebral bodies result from failure of fusion of anterior and posterior ossification centres, and are also seen in metatropic dwarfism and Kniest syndrome.

b) **False** Hurler's syndrome is associated with beaks from the lower third of the vertebral body, as are achondroplasia, pseudoachondroplasia, hypothyroidism, Down's syndrome and neuromuscular diseases. Morquio's syndrome is associated with central beaks.

c) **True** Diffuse platyspondyly is also seen in thanatophoric and metatropic dwarfism, Morquio's syndrome, Kniest syndrome and spondyloepiphyseal dysplasia (congenita and tarda).

d) **True** A solitary ivory vertebral body occurs less commonly in non-Hodgkin's lymphoma, and is also seen with sclerotic metastases, Paget's disease, haemangioma and chronic infection.

e) **True** Deafness is seen in about 30% of Klippel–Feil syndrome cases. Other nonspinal features include renal agenesis in 33% of cases and congenital heart disease (atrial septal defect and coarctation) in 5% of cases.

40 a) **True** A Jefferson fracture results from an axial compression force transmitted through the vertex to the axis, causing lateral displacement (hence it tends to spare the cord) of lateral masses and fractures of anterior and posterior arches of C1.

   b) **False** The flexion teardrop fracture is a severely unstable injury resulting from flexion fracture–dislocation, which presents with acute anterior cord dysfunction. All ligaments are disrupted and a combination of posterior vertebral body subluxation and bilateral facet joint subluxation/dislocation compromises the adjacent cord. This injury should not to be confused with the stable extension teardrop fracture.

   c) **True** Chance fractures are produced by hyperflexion secondary to falls or vehicular accidents whilst wearing a seatbelt. There is distraction and disruption of the posterior and middle columns. There is a 20% chance of neurological or abdominal organ injury.

   d) **True** This indicates haemorrhage, which has a very poor prognosis, unlike oedema of the cord (high signal on T2-weighted imaging), which offers a good potential for recovery.

   e) **False** Nerve root avulsions are usually caused by traction injuries to the extremities, hence they spare the thoracic spine. Complete avulsions lead to CSF-filled pseudomeningocoeles.

Chapter 7

Head and neck imaging

1   **Which of the following are true of head and neck imaging?**
   a)   The prevertebral space extends from the base of the skull to the diaphragm
   b)   The parapharyngeal space typically has high signal on T1-weighted magnetic resonance imaging (MRI)
   c)   The pterygopalatine fossa communicates with the middle cranial fossa
   d)   The facial nerve within the parotid gland runs lateral to the retromandibular vein
   e)   The masticator space communicates with the middle cranial fossa

2   **Regarding Tornwaldt's cysts, which of the following are true?**
   a)   They are midline in location
   b)   They do not enhance after contrast on computed tomography (CT)
   c)   They are usually low signal on T1-weighted MRI sequence
   d)   They erode bone
   e)   They typically arise caudal to Rathke's pouch cyst

3   **Which of the following are true of sinonasal imaging?**
   a)   The ostiomeatal complex is best evaluated in the coronal plane
   b)   Haller cells are the most posterior extensions of the ethmoid air cells
   c)   Mucocoeles most commonly involve the sphenoidal sinus
   d)   Meningoencephalocoele is a recognised complication of funduscopic endonasal sinus surgery
   e)   Squamous cell carcinoma accounts for 80% of malignancies of the paranasal sinus

4   **Concerning thyroglossal duct cysts, which of the following are true?**
   a)   The majority occur above the level of the hyoid bone
   b)   About 90% of cases present before 5 years of age
   c)   Ultrasound or radionuclide study is indicated prior to surgical excision
   d)   Capsular enhancement on CT indicates infection
   e)   Carcinoma is a rare complication

5   **Which of the following are true regarding haemangioma of the head and neck?**
   a)   They are the most common benign tumours of the head and neck in the first few years of life
   b)   About 50% of cutaneous haemangiomas resolve by 5 years of age
   c)   Intramuscularly, haemangiomas of the head and neck most commonly involve sternocleidomastoid muscles
   d)   Haemangiomas may be distinguished from lymphangiomas by technetium-labelled red blood cell study
   e)   They typically show intermediate signal on T1-weighted MRI and heterogeneously high signal on T2-weighted MRI

6   **Which of the following are true regarding dermoid and epidermoid cysts?**
   a)   The most common location of dermoid cyst in the head and neck is the orbit
   b)   High signal on T1-weighted MRI is diagnostic of a dermoid cyst
   c)   Dermoid cysts may be distinguished from lipoma on T1-weighted MRI
   d)   Epidermoid cysts are usually unilocular
   e)   Epidermoid cysts have high signal on T2-weighted MRI scans

7   **Which of the following are true regarding laryngocoeles?**
   a) They typically arise in the vestibule
   b) They are bilateral in less than 5% of cases
   c) They may appear as hypodense masses on unenhanced CT
   d) Carcinoma is a recognised complication
   e) They rarely extend beyond the thyrohyoid membrane

8   **Which of the following are true regarding the salivary gland?**
   a) There is an increased risk of lymphoma of the parotid gland in Sjögren's syndrome
   b) Warthin's tumour of the parotid gland is bilateral in 10% of cases
   c) About 50% of minor salivary gland tumours are malignant
   d) Mucoepidermoid carcinoma is the most common malignant tumour of the parotid gland
   e) Through-transmission is a typical feature of pleomorphic salivary gland adenoma

9   **Which of the following are true of head and neck imaging?**
   a) Cervical lipomas most commonly occur in the posterior triangle of the neck
   b) Paragangliomas are hypervascular lesions
   c) Ranulas are usually high signal on T1- and T2-weighted MRI
   d) Second branchial cleft cysts are typically located anteromedial to the sternocleidomastoid muscle
   e) Melanomas demonstrate shortening of T1- and T2-weighted values on MRI

10 **Concerning imaging of the larynx, which of the following are true?**
   a) The arytenoids usually dislocate rather than fracture during trauma
   b) Cricoid cartilage typically fractures in at least two places following trauma
   c) More than 90% of laryngeal cancers are squamous cell tumours
   d) Glottic cancers typically arise from the anterior half of the vocal cord
   e) At presentation, subglottic tumours are frequently nonoperative

11 **Which of the following are true regarding juvenile angiofibromas?**
   a) They are highly vascular
   b) They extend into the pterygopalatine fossa in more than 90% of cases
   c) They typically displace the posterior wall of the maxillary sinus
   d) They may cause widening of the superior and inferior orbital fissure
   e) They show areas of low signal on T1-weighted MRI

12 **Which of the following are true concerning parathyroid imaging?**
   a) Supernumerary glands are found in at least 25% of patients
   b) Primary hyperparathyroidism is caused by a single hyperfunctioning adenoma in 80% of cases
   c) Parathyroid adenomas characteristically return high signal on T2-weighted images
   d) About 10% of parathyroid glands are found in the mediastinum
   e) On CT, 50% of adenomas typically enhance after intravenous contrast

13 **Regarding thyroid carcinoma, which of the following are true?**
   a) Follicular carcinoma accounts for 60% of all thyroid carcinomas
   b) Lymph node spread occurs in 90% of patients with papillary cell carcinoma
   c) Early haematogenous spread occurs in follicular carcinoma
   d) Anaplastic carcinoma demonstrates no radioiodine uptake
   e) Multiple endocrine neoplasia (MEN) type IIb may be associated with medullary cell carcinoma

14 **Which of the following are true regarding laryngeal carcinoma?**
   a) Most are supraglottic in location
   b) Supraglottic carcinomas usually present later than glottic cancer
   c) The normal anterior commissure should be no thicker than 1 mm
   d) About 50% of subglottic cancers involve the thyroid or cricoid cartilage
   e) Cartilage invasion implies T4 disease

15 **Which of the following are true regarding facial fractures?**
   a) Orbital fractures are the most common fractures of the facial skeleton
   b) All Le Fort fractures involve the pterygoid plates
   c) Le Fort fractures are usually associated with fractures of the zygomaticomaxillary complex
   d) In blunt trauma, isolated medial wall fractures of the orbit are common
   e) An intact orbital rim is typical of an orbital blow-out fracture

16 **Regarding imaging of the ear, which of the following are true?**
   a) Limited hearing is possible with a Michel aplasia
   b) Cholesteatomas are hyperintense on T1- and T2-weighted images
   c) Ossicular chain disruption is a feature of cholesterol granulomas
   d) The normal vestibular aqueduct may be up to 5 mm in diameter
   e) Otosclerosis most commonly involves the stapes

17 **Regarding trauma to the ear, which of the following are true?**
   a) The most common cause of conductive deafness following head injury is ossicular chain disruption
   b) Most fractures of the petrous bone are longitudinal
   c) Longitudinal fractures of the petrous bone are usually associated with sensorineural deafness
   d) The facial nerve is involved in 50% of transverse fractures of the petrous bone
   e) The most common site of ossicular injury is the incudostapedial junction

18 **Which of the following are true regarding perineural spread of head and neck tumours?**
   a) Enhancement of the nerve is a reliable sign of perineural spread
   b) The nerve most commonly involved in perineural spread of head and neck tumours is the facial nerve
   c) Loss of high T1-weighted MRI signal in the pterygopalatine fossa is a sign of perineural spread of the tumour
   d) Adenoid cystic carcinoma is one of the most common tumours to show perineural spread
   e) Acutely denervated muscle typically returns high T2-weighted MRI signal

19 Which of the following are true regarding sarcomas of the head and neck?
 a) Rhabdomyosarcomas typically occur in patients over the age of 40 years
 b) The most common site of rhabdomyosarcomas in the head and neck is the nasopharynx
 c) Fibrosarcoma of the head and neck usually involves the mandible and maxilla
 d) Leiomyosarcomas of the head and neck usually involve the sinonasal cavity
 e) Liposarcomas typically have high signal on T1-weighted MRI sequences

20 Which of the following are true of the salivary glands?
 a) Malignant tumours of the salivary glands are more common than benign lesions
 b) Adenoid cystic carcinoma most commonly affects the submandibular gland
 c) About 80% of parotid gland tumours arise in the superficial part of the gland
 d) Pleomorphic adenomas of the parotid gland typically have high signal on T2-weighted MRI sequences
 e) The normal parotid gland contains lymph nodes

21 Which of the following are true of fibrous dysplasia?
 a) Facial bones are rarely involved
 b) Exophthalmos is a recognised feature
 c) There is an association with Cushing's syndrome
 d) In the calvaria, the frontal bone is most commonly involved
 e) It affects the maxilla more frequently than the mandible

22 Which of the following cause loss of the lamina dura of the teeth?
 a) Hyperparathyroidism
 b) Cushing's disease
 c) Addison's disease
 d) Paget's disease
 e) Sickle cell disease

23 Which of the following are true regarding lesions of the jaw?
 a) Ameloblastoma occurs more frequently in the maxilla
 b) A dentigerous cyst develops around an unerupted tooth
 c) Dentigerous cysts are associated with basal cell naevi
 d) Radicular cysts arise in relation to the tooth apex
 e) Simple bone cysts are more common in the maxilla than the mandible

24 Which of the following are true regarding trauma to the neck?
 a) In blunt neck trauma, dissection of the extracranial carotid artery is asymptomatic in 10% of cases
 b) Multiple levels are involved in 20% of fractures of the cervical spine
 c) The most common site of vertebral artery injury in blunt trauma to the neck is at the C5/C6 level
 d) Fracture of the odontoid peg most commonly involves the tip
 e) Barium swallow has poor sensitivity for pharyngoesophageal injury in blunt neck trauma

25 **Which of the following are true regarding Klippel–Feil syndrome?**
   a) It is associated with Sprengel's shoulder deformity
   b) Conductive hearing loss is a feature
   c) Vertebral fusion involves the bodies and neural arches
   d) Coarctation is a feature
   e) Lymphoedema is a feature

26 **Which of the following are true regarding imaging of the thyroid gland?**
   a) ^{131}I is the preferred agent in thyroid gland imaging
   b) Most cold nodules are neoplastic
   c) About 25% of solitary nodules on scintigraphy are multinodular on ultrasonography
   d) Cold nodules on scintigraphy are usually hyperechoic on ultrasonography
   e) Focal thyroiditis is a recognised cause of a cold nodule on scintigraphy

27 **Which of the following are true of laryngeal papillomatosis?**
   a) There is a bimodal age distribution
   b) The lung is involved in 5% of cases
   c) Subglottic extension is rarely seen
   d) There is an association with bronchiectasis
   e) Malignant transformation is a recognised complication

28 **Which of the following are true regarding 2-[^{18}F]-fluoro-2-deoxy-D-glucose (FDG) positron emission tomography (PET) in head and neck imaging?**
   a) FDG competes with glucose for uptake
   b) High FDG uptake is seen in the normal lingual tonsils
   c) A standardised uptake value (SUV) greater than 3.5 for cervical lymph nodes suggests malignancy
   d) FDG PET is highly specific for malignant thyroid nodules
   e) A decrease in FDG uptake shortly after radiotherapy indicates disease response

29 **Which of the following are true regarding the carotid artery?**
   a) The carotid bulb is the most common part of the carotid artery to be affected by atherosclerotic disease
   b) Ultrasound can accurately identify ulcerated atherosclerotic plaques
   c) Multiple stenosis of the carotid artery is seen in up to 20% of cases
   d) Fibromuscular dysplasia of the carotid artery most commonly involves the artery below the bulb
   e) Carotid artery dissection related to trauma usually commences at the origin of the internal carotid artery

30 **Which of the following are true regarding fractures of the cervical spine?**
   a) Flexion teardrop fractures involve the superior endplate of the vertebral body
   b) Clay shoveler's fracture is stable
   c) In bilateral interfacetal dislocation, there is anterior translocation of the involved vertebra by at least 50% of the diameter of the subjacent vertebrae
   d) Hangman's fracture is a bilateral fracture of the neural arches of C2
   e) Unilateral interfacet joint dislocation is a stable injury

31 Which of the following are true regarding cholesteatomas?
a) The majority are congenital
b) Acquired cholesteatoma is associated with a disrupted tympanic membrane
c) They arise from Prussak's space
d) They typically enhance with gadolinium
e) Labyrinthine fistulae are a recognised complication

32 Which of the following are true of the oral cavity?
a) Squamous cell carcinoma accounts for 90% of malignant tumours of the oral cavity
b) Pleomorphic adenomas are the most common benign glandular tumours of the oral cavity
c) Squamous cell carcinoma of the oral tongue spreads to the submandibular lymph nodes
d) The most common site of squamous cell carcinoma in the oral cavity is the mucosa of the upper lip
e) Ranulas frequently present as bilateral masses in the floor of the mouth

33 Which of the following are true regarding salivary gland calculi?
a) More than 80% of salivary gland stones occur in the submandibular gland
b) About 25% of patients have multiple stones
c) Most submandibular stones are radio-opaque
d) Submandibular stones typically occur within Wharton's duct
e) Asymptomatic intraductal parotid stones can be an incidental finding on CT

34 Which of the following are true regarding imaging of the lacrimal system?
a) The most common site of obstruction is at the distal end of the nasolacrimal duct
b) Lacrimal duct calculi are present in up to 30% of patients with chronic dacryocystitis
c) Diverticula of the nasolacrimal duct are usually the result of obstruction
d) Fistulae of the nasolacrimal system typically involve the lacrimal sac
e) Dacryoscintigraphy (DSG) is more sensitive at detecting obstruction than contrast dacryocystography (DCG)

35 Which of the following are true of tumours of the skull base?
a) Chordomas in the clivus commonly present with nasopharyngeal obstruction
b) Chordomas typically enhance after contrast
c) Meningiomas cause widening of sutures
d) Chondrosarcomas at the skull base are usually related to the synchondrosis or fissures
e) Secondary involvement of the skull base is usually by haematogenous spread

36 Which of the following are true regarding imaging of the brachial plexus?
a) Coronal MRI sequences are useful
b) 50% of brachial plexus injuries result from trauma
c) Brachial plexopathy postradiotherapy typically presents within 1 year of treatment
d) In patients with brachial plexopathy, MRI is useful in distinguishing tumour recurrence from postradiotherapy change
e) Brachial plexus avulsion injuries are accurately diagnosed by myelography

37 Which of the following are true regarding imaging of lymphoma of the head and neck?
   a) In Hodgkin's disease, Waldeyer's ring is typically spared
   b) Extranodal involvement is common in non-Hodgkin's lymphoma
   c) Lymph nodes involved in Hodgkin's disease typically show homogenous contrast enhancement
   d) Lymph node calcification is common before treatment
   e) Lymphoma of the orbit most commonly involves the optic nerve sheath

38 Which of the following are true regarding granulocytic sarcoma (chloroma)?
   a) It typically affects children
   b) It usually presents as a solitary lesion
   c) It is associated with myeloproliferative disease in up to 50% of patients
   d) It typically enhances after contrast on CT
   e) It rarely involves the paranasal sinuses

39 Which of the following are true regarding the facial nerve?
   a) The facial nerve lies within the anterosuperior quadrant of the internal auditory canal
   b) The facial nerve may protrude through the oval window
   c) Facial nerve neuroma is the most common cause of hemifacial spasm
   d) The most common neoplasm of the VII nerve is a schwannoma
   e) Mild enhancement of the facial nerve on MRI is suggestive of an underlying inflammatory/infectious process

40 Which of the following are true regarding cross-sectional imaging of the head and neck?
   a) The carotid sheath lies posterior to the styloid process
   b) The carotid sheath normally contains lymph nodes
   c) Neuroblastoma is the most common primary carotid sheath malignancy in children
   d) The presence of flow voids in a mass greater than 2 cm involving the carotid artery favours a diagnosis of a paraganglioma rather than a schwannoma
   e) The most common lesion of the carotid sheath is a paraganglioma

Answers

1 a) **True**   The retropharyngeal space lies posterior to the parapharyngeal space and medial to the carotid space, and is divided into anterior and posterior compartments by fascia. The posterior compartment, which is also known as the prevertebral space, extends from the skull base through the mediastinum to the diaphragm. This allows infection to track down into the posterior mediastinum.

    b) **True**   This is the major space in the suprahyoid neck and contains mostly fat, but also major vessels, ectopic minor salivary rest cells and lymph nodes. Displacement of the fat in the parapharyngeal space helps to localise lesions.

    c) **True**   The pterygopalatine fossa communicates with the paranasal sinuses, masticator space, nasopharynx, orbit and middle cranial fossa via the foramen rotundum, hence the importance in the spread of disease. It contains the pterygopalatine ganglion and maxillary nerve.

    d) **True**   The normal nerve may not be seen on MRI; hence, the position may be inferred from the vein.

    e) **True**   Perineural spread of the tumour can occur via the foramen ovale into the middle cranial fossa.

2 a) **True**   Tornwaldt's cysts arise as a result of focal adhesion between the ectoderm and regressing notochord. This forms a small pouch. When the connection with the pouch is closed, a cyst results.

    b) **True**   They are well-defined, nonenhancing cysts between the prevertebral muscles in the posterior roof of the nasopharynx.

    c) **False**   Protein in the cyst increases T1 value, thus increasing the signal on T1-weighted scans.

    d) **False**   They do not cause bone erosion. They are rarely calcified and usually hypodense on CT.

    e) **True**   Rathke's pouch cysts are located anterior and cephalad to Tornwaldt's cysts.

3 a) **True**   The anterior ostiomeatal complex consists of the maxillary sinus ostium, infundibulum, uncinate process, hiatus semilunaris, ethmoidal bullae, middle turbinate and meatus. It is best evaluated on direct coronal scanning.

    b) **False**   Haller cells are the most anterior of the ethmoid air cells. They predispose to sinus disease.

    c) **False**   Mucocoeles are expansile lesions, which arise secondary to occlusion of the sinus ostium. They most frequently affect the frontal sinus (65% of cases) followed by the ethmoid sinus. The sphenoid sinus is rarely involved.

    d) **True**   Other complications recognised on CT include orbital trauma (haematoma, lamina papyracea disruption, surgical emphysema, abscess, orbital nerve damage) and intracranial injury (pneumocephalus, cerebrospinal fluid [CSF] leak, haematoma, cerebritis, abscess). The most common site of injury is the lateral lamella.

    e) **True**   Squamous cell carcinoma affects the maxillary sinus in 80% of cases. Other malignancies include adenocarcinoma, adenoid cystic carcinoma and sarcoma.

4 a) **False** About 65% arise below, 15% at and 20% above the level of the hyoid bone.
     b) **False** About 30% are diagnosed after age 20 years. Failure of involution of the thyroglossal duct, which extends from the foramen caecum to the thyroid gland in the neck, may result in a cyst anywhere along its course. The infrahyoid cysts are often paramedian. Suprahyoid cysts are midline.
     c) **True** It is important to confirm the presence of functioning thyroid tissue before surgery.
     d) **False** Thyroglossal duct cysts are typically unilocular with capsular enhancement. Enhancement does not necessarily indicate infection. Features of infection may include thickened overlying skin and platysma.
     e) **True** Carcinoma is a complication in less than 1% of all cases. Infection is much more common.

5 a) **True** They are the most common benign tumour of infancy. Haemangiomas are true benign neoplasms, which increase in size in the first few years of life.
     b) **True** They are also three times more common in females than males.
     c) **False** Intramuscular haemangiomas involve the posterior triangle muscles – trapezius and masseter.
     d) **True** However, this is frequently unnecessary in clinical practice.
     e) **True** They are typically isointense with muscle on T1-weighted MRI and hyperintense on T2-weighted MRI. They enhance briskly with contrast and may show multiple flow voids.

6 a) **True** Common sites of dermoid cysts are lateral margins of the orbit, and the oral and nasal cavities. Oral cavity lesions present later.
     b) **False** Fat with high T1 signal is seen in other lesions (e.g. lipoma). Dermoid cysts are usually hyperintense on T1-weighted MRI and isointense with muscle on T2-weighted MRI.
     c) **False** Both may contain fat, which has a high signal on T1-weighted imaging.
     d) **True** Epidermoid cysts are inclusions of epidermal elements. They are usually unilocular and thin walled.
     e) **True** Epidermoid cysts are usually hypointense on T1-weighted imaging and hyperintense on T2-weighted imaging.

7 a) **False** They arise at the saccule of the ventricle, secondary to obstruction of the laryngeal ventricles. Occasionally this is due to cancer.
     b) **False** They are bilateral in 25% of cases.
     c) **True** They may contain air or fluid.
     d) **True** Carcinoma occurs in less than 1% of cases. Other complications include infection or mucocoele formation.
     e) **False** In relation to the thyrohyoid membrane, 30% are internal, 26% are external and 44% are mixed.

8 a) **True** There is a 44-fold increased risk of non-Hodgkin's lymphoma.
     b) **True** Other bilateral tumours include acinus cell tumour and lymphoma.
     c) **True** This is associated with a poor prognosis.
     d) **True** Mucoepidermoid carcinoma presents as a hard mass, which may be low grade (well defined) or high grade (with an infiltrating edge).
     e) **True** The ultrasound features of pleomorphic salivary gland adenoma are classical: a hypoechoic, lobulated mass with through transmission.

9 a) **True** Lipomas are encapsulated masses of mature fat found mostly in the posterior triangle.

b) **True** Paragangliomas (glomus jugulare, glomus vagale and carotid body tumours) are hypervascular lesions. MRI may show flow voids.

c) **False** Ranulas are retention cysts in the submucosal gland. They are high signal on T2-weighted scans and may have low, iso, or high signal on T1-weighted scans.

d) **True** However, they may be seen anywhere along the course of the developing second branchial cleft (tonsillar fossa to the supraclavicular fossa) and classically extend between the internal and external carotid arteries.

e) **True** This is due to the paramagnetic properties of melanin. They are high signal on T1-weighted scans and low on T2-weighted MRI.

10 a) **True** Following trauma, the arytenoids dislocate anteriorly and superiorly.

b) **True** Cricoid cartilage is a ring structure and fractures in at least two places.

c) **True** Squamous carcinoma is supraglottic in 20%–30% of cases, glottic in 50%–60% and subglottic in only 5% of cases.

d) **True** Tumours may then spread into the anterior commissure from where they can spread to the supraglottic and subglottic region.

e) **True** Subglottic tumours are rare. They usually represent extension of glottic tumours. They may then invade the trachea, oesophagus and thyroid. They have a poor prognosis due to late presentation and detection.

11 All true Juvenile angiofibromas most commonly occur in teenage males. They are highly vascular and arise in the posterior nares and nasopharynx. They extend into the pterygopalatine fossa in more than 90% of cases and can involve the middle cranial fossa and orbit, causing widening of the superior and inferior orbital fissure. Biopsy is contraindicated because of the risk of bleeding. CT shows immediate enhancement after intravenous contrast and MRI shows intermediate signal on T1-weighted imaging, with focal areas of low signal due to signal voids. Presurgical embolisation can be considered.

12 a) **True**

b) **True** About 15% of cases are caused by parathyroid hyperplasia and 1% by hyperfunctioning parathyroid carcinoma.

c) **False** However, 25% show high signal on T2-weighted MRI.

d) **True** About 20% of glands are ectopic and 10% are found within the mediastinum.

e) **False** About 25% of adenomas enhance on CT. However, detection largely depends on adenoma size. Power Doppler may show increased vascularity.

13 a) **False**   Papillary carcinoma accounts for 60%, follicular 20%, anaplastic 4%–15% and medullary 1%–5%.

b) **False**   Papillary carcinoma metastasises to nodes in 40% of adult cases (but 90% of child cases). Haematogenous spread is much less common. It affects the lungs in 4% of cases and rarely bone.

c) **True**   Follicular carcinoma shows early haematogenous spread to lung and bone.

d) **True**   Papillary carcinoma usually takes up radioiodine. Follicular carcinoma concentrates pertechnetate but not iodine (^{123}I). Medullary carcinoma demonstrates no iodine or pertechnetate uptake, but does concentrate thallium (^{201}Tl).

e) **True**   Medullary carcinoma may be associated with MEN IIa (phaeochromocytoma, hyperparathyroidism and medullary carcinoma) and MEN IIb (phaeochromocytoma, medullary carcinoma, oral and intestinal ganglioneuromas and a marfanoid habitus).

14 a) **False**   Most are glottic carcinomas (50%–60%); supraglottic carcinoma accounts for 20%–30% and subglottic carcinoma 5% of cases.

b) **True**   Glottic carcinoma presents early with hoarseness. Supraglottic carcinoma presents late (typically T3/T4 disease) and 50% have lymphadenopathy.

c) **True**   Thickening of the anterior commissure greater than 1 mm is suspicious of tumour involvement.

d) **True**   Subglottic cancer presents late and spreads circumferentially. Almost 50% of cases will involve the cricoid or thyroid cartilage. Inferior spread may involve the trachea.

e) **True**   Cartilage involvement indicates T4 disease and often precludes conservative surgery. Cartilage involvement is largely related to tumour size and site and not to histology. It is best assessed with MRI.

15 a) **False**   Nasal fractures are the most common facial bone fractures.

b) **True**   Le Fort I is a transverse fracture through the maxilla. Le Fort II involves a fracture through the alveolar ridge, medial orbital rim and nasal bone. Le Fort III involves a fracture through the nasofrontal suture, frontomaxillary suture, orbital wall and zygomatic arch and results in craniofacial instability.

c) **True**   There is usually an associated zygomaticomaxillary complex fracture on the side of the trauma. To sustain a true Le Fort fracture, the face must be exactly perpendicular to the force of impact.

d) **False**   The medial wall of the orbit is commonly fractured in an orbital blow-out fracture in which the floor is also fractured. An isolated medial wall fracture is uncommon and usually results from penetrating trauma.

e) **True**   Other radiographic features of blow-out orbital fracture include: soft tissue projecting from the floor of the orbit into the maxillary sinus, a depressed fragment of orbital floor hanging obliquely from medial to lateral, and opacification of the maxillary sinus.

16 a) **False**   A Michel aplasia is total aplasia of the inner ear. The Mondini deformity preserves the basal turn of the cochlea, allowing some hearing.

   b) **False**   Cholesteatomas are isointense to brain on T1-weighted imaging and hyperintense on T2-weighted imaging. (Compare this with cholesterol granulomas, which are hyperintense on both T1- and T2-weighted imaging.) There is no enhancement following intravenous gadolinium.

   c) **False**   Cholesteatomas are a focal collection of exfoliated keratin within a sac of squamous epithelium. They may be acquired or, rarely, congenital. They may erode the tegmen tympani, cause labyrinthine fistula and disrupt the ossicular chain (initially the long process of the incus).

   d) **False**   A vestibular aqueduct larger than 2 mm is abnormal. Vestibular aqueduct syndrome can present with unilateral congenital deafness and is commonly missed radiologically.

   e) **True**   Otosclerosis involves the stapes in 80%–90% of cases. There is progressive bone formation at the oval window with fixation of the stapes. This is bilateral in 90% of cases.

17 a) **False**   The most common cause of deafness after head injury is haemotympanum or rupture of the ear drum.

   b) **True**   About 75% of fractures are longitudinal and parallel to the long axis of the petrous bone.

   c) **False**   Longitudinal fractures usually result in conductive deafness due to disruption of the ossicular chain, especially the incus. Facial nerve palsy is seen in only 10%–20% of cases. This is usually due to oedema and recovers spontaneously.

   d) **True**   With transverse fractures, spontaneous recovery is less common than with longitudinal fractures. If the fracture line crosses the apex of the petrous temporal bone with involvement of the internal auditory canal and labyrinth, then irreversible sensorineural hearing loss will result.

   e) **True**   This joint is poorly demonstrated on cross-sectional imaging.

18 a) **False**   Enhancement may be seen with normal nerves due to the presence of perineural vascular plexus.

   b) **False**   The trigeminal nerve is the largest cranial nerve and the most common nerve involved in perineural spread.

   c) **True**   Loss of perineural fat in the pterygopalatine fossa is a useful indicator of perineural spread along the V2 branches of the trigeminal nerve. In addition to loss of fat planes adjacent to nerves, other signs include: erosion or enlargement of nerve foramina, and enlargement and abnormal enhancement of the nerve with loss of distinction between the nerve and its perineural vascular plexus.

   d) **True**   Common tumours to show perineural spread include squamous cell tumour and adenoid cystic tumour of the salivary gland.

   e) **True**   Denervation is a feature of perineural spread. Denervated muscle returns high T2 signal acutely. Chronic changes include fatty replacement and atrophy.

19 a) **False** 78% occur under the age of 12 years. A second peak is seen between ages 15 and 19 years.

b) **False** The most frequent sites of origin of rhabdomyosarcomas are the head and neck (43%), genitourinary system (29%), trunk (16%) and extremities. The most common sites in the head and neck are the orbit (36%), nasopharynx (15%), middle ear and mastoid.

c) **True** 15% of fibrosarcomas involve the head and neck, usually the maxilla, mandible, sinonasal cavity and larynx. The typical age group is 30–50 years.

d) **True** Leiomyosarcomas arise from smooth muscle. Up to 10% involve the head and neck, and usually the sinonasal cavity. The typical age of occurrence is 50 years. They are bulky tumours, which have areas of cystic and necrotic change.

e) **True** The usual age of onset of liposarcomas is 40 years and 3% involve the head and neck, where they usually involve the sinonasal cavity and soft tissues of the neck.

20 a) **False** Malignant tumours are less common than benign tumours. They are usually adenoid cystic or mucoepidermoid tumours.

b) **False** It comprises 30% of malignant neoplasms of the minor salivary glands, 15% of submandibular tumours and 2%–6% of parotid gland tumours. The 10-year survival rate is 40%. Adenoid cystic tumour is a malignant tumour, which shows early perineural spread along the facial nerve.

c) **True** About 80% of salivary gland tumours arise in the parotid gland and 80% of parotid tumours arise in the superficial lobe. A total of 80% of parotid tumors are benign.

d) **True** Pleomorphic adenomas comprise 70% of parotid tumours, show high T2 signal, and are usually well defined. They are mostly seen in women over 60 years of age.

e) **True** However, nodal enlargement is usually due to infection, inflammation, or metastases.

21 a) **False** Fibrous dysplasia typically presents before the age of 30 years. The most common sites of involvement are the ribs (30%), cranium and facial bones (25%) and femur and tibia (25%).

b) **True** Other head and neck manifestations include cranial asymmetry, visual impairment due to foraminal narrowing, and cranial and orbital asymmetry. Extensive craniofacial involvement may result in leontiasis ossea.

c) **True** Other associations include precocious puberty in girls with café-au-lait spots (McCune–Albright syndrome), hyperthyroidism, hyperparathyroidism, acromegaly and diabetes mellitus.

d) **True** The most common sites in the skull are the frontal bone, sphenoid and, less commonly, hemicranial involvement.

e) **True** In the maxilla, it typically causes a localised homogenous opacity with an increase in size on one side.

22 a) **True**
b) **True**
c) **False**
d) **True**
e) **False**

Other causes of loss of the lamina dura include osteoporosis, osteomalacia, scleroderma, localised infection and metastasis/leukaemia.

23 a) **False**   About 75% of ameloblastomas arise in the mandible, usually at the angle. They may be multilocular and are cystic expansile lesions, which often recur after excision.

  b) **True**   Dentigerous cysts arise adjacent to an unerupted crown, usually a wisdom/canine tooth. They may be multilocular.

  c) **True**   Gorlin's syndrome comprises dentigerous cysts, multiple basal cell naevi, rib anomalies and falx calcification. Medulloblastomas may also be seen in children. It has an autosomal dominant inheritance.

  d) **True**   Radicular cysts are common benign cystic lesions near the apex of a caries tooth, which may erode into the mandible, displacing adjacent teeth.

  e) **False**   Bone cysts are unilocular and well defined. They may be trauma-related and typically arise in the body of the mandible.

24 a) **False**   Dissection of the extracranial carotid artery is asymptomatic at presentation in 50% of cases. Diagnosis may be delayed.

  b) **True**   C2 is the most common fracture site, followed by C6 and C5. The posterior elements are fractured in over 50% of cases and the body is involved in 30% of cervical spine fractures. The thoracic and lumbar spine may be involved in 15%–20% of cases.

  c) **False**   Vertebral artery injury is usually due to stretching and occurs most frequently at the C1/C2 level. Vertebral artery injuries are more common than carotid artery injuries in blunt neck trauma.

  d) **False**   Odontoid peg fractures are divided into three types. Type 1 is a fracture of the tip (5%–8%). Type 2 is a fracture at the base (54%–67%). Type 3 is a subodontoid peg fracture (30%–33%).

  e) **False**   Barium swallow and endoscopy have 89% and 94% sensitivity for pharyngoesophageal injury, respectively, with nearly 100% specificity.

25 a) **True**   Other associations include syringomyelia, platybasia, clubbed foot, hemivertebrae and congenital heart disease (e.g. coarctation). One third have renal agenesis.

  b) **True**   Deafness occurs in 30% of cases and can be due to an absent auditory canal, and ossicular and labyrinthine maldevelopment.

  c) **True**   Fusion may involve the craniovertebral junction and cervicothoracic junction.
  d) **True**
  e) **True**

26 a) **False** ^{123}I is preferred mainly due to its 159 keV γ energy, short half-life and low radiation dose. ^{131}I has a higher radiation dose and can be used for the treatment of functioning thyroid cancer.

  b) **False**   Only 5%–20% of cold nodules on scintigraphy are neoplastic.
  c) **True**

  d) **False**   Cold nodules on scintigraphy are usually hypoechoic on ultrasound scanning. Less commonly, they are isoechoic and, rarely, hyperechoic (3%).

  e) **True**   Other causes of cold nodule include carcinoma, lymphoma, granuloma, abscess, cyst and parathyroid tumour.

27 a) **True** Laryngeal papillomatosis consists of benign squamous papillomas, which may be single or diffuse. They typically affect those under 10 or 20–50 years old. The latter group usually have a single papilloma.

b) **True** Presentation includes hoarseness, stridor, recurrent infection and haemoptysis.

c) **False** Areas of involvement include the uvula and palate, vocal cords and subglottic extension (50%–70% of cases).

d) **True** Complications include: pulmonary involvement, tracheobronchial papilloma and bronchiectasis.

e) **True** This is usually squamous cell carcinoma.

28 a) **True** FDG PET depends on altered metabolic activity of tumour tissue, in particular increased glycolysis. FDG is a glucose analogue, which competes with native glucose and becomes trapped within tumour cells with increased glycolysis. Patients are fasted for 6 hours before the FDG injection. Diabetics should have their glucose normalised before injection.

b) **True** Normal physiological uptake is seen in the cerebellar hemispheres and temporal lobes and milder uptake occurs in the cervical spinal cord. The highest activity is seen in the palatine and lingual tonsils, lips and sublingual glands.

c) **True** SUV is a semiquantitative method of evaluating FDG uptake. It is derived by the following equation: SUV = decay corrected tissue activity concentration in the tumour ÷ injected dose/body weight. SUV of cervical metastatic nodes ranges 2–11 with a mean of 3.7. As benign inflammatory nodes have a reported SUV up to 15.8, there is overlap. However, an SUV larger than 3.5 may be considered to indicate malignancy, especially when the PET findings are interpreted together with the results of clinical examination and other imaging methods.

d) **True** FDG PET is highly sensitive and specific. However, it does not indicate whether the tumour cells will take up ^{131}I. FDG PET is mainly indicated in the posttherapy setting when the carcinoma is less differentiated and more metabolically active. Patients with less well-differentiated carcinoma are less able to concentrate radioiodine. PET is also useful in patients with Hürthle cell carcinoma, anaplastic thyroid cancers and in the detection of metastases or minimal residual disease in those with medullary carcinoma of the thyroid.

e) **False** After radiotherapy, FDG uptake may decrease markedly, but remain stable in normal tissue. In order to avoid these false-positive and later false-negative results, FDG PET should not be undertaken within 4 months of radiotherapy.

29 a) **True** Atherosclerosis typically involves the posterior-lateral aspect of the bulb in the early stages.

b) **False** Ulcerated plaques are prone to platelet aggregation and embolus. The best technique to diagnose an ulcerated plaque is angiography (sensitivity 46% and specificity 74%).

c) **True** Multiple stenoses are seen in 20% of cases and most commonly involve the cavernous segment of the internal carotid artery (ICA). This area is poorly imaged by magnetic resonance angiography.

d) **False** Fibromuscular dysplasia affects the ICA above the level of the bulb; it typically affects women (F:M = 9:1) aged 50–70 years.

e) **False** Carotid dissection causes 20% of strokes in those less than 40 years old. When related to trauma, the site of origin is usually the ICA at the level of the C2 vertebral body.

30 a) **False** Flexion teardrop fractures involve avulsion of the anterior inferior corner, usually of the C2 vertebral body with displacement of the involved vertebral body into the spinal column. There is disruption of all soft-tissue structures with an associated acute anterior cervical cord syndrome.

b) **True** This is an oblique fracture of the spinous process of C6, C7 or T1.

c) **True** In bilateral interfacetal joint dislocation, the articular masses of the involved vertebra dislocate and rest anterior to the superior facets of the subjacent vertebrae.

d) **True** This is associated with anterior subluxation of C2 on C3.

e) **True** The involved inferior articulating facet of the vertebra above is dislocated anterior to the superior facet of the vertebra below.

31 a) **False** 98% are acquired. Cholesteatomas represent exfoliated keratin within a squamous epithelium sac.

b) **True** Cholesteatomas are associated with marginal perforation of the tympanic membrane and chronic mastoiditis.

c) **True** Acquired cholesteatomas are thought to arise from retraction pockets in the superior pars flaccida of the tympanic membrane within Prussak's space. This space is located between the malleus neck and the lateral wall of the attic.

d) **False** No enhancement is seen following intravenous gadolinium.

e) **True** Fistulae usually occur at the level of the lateral semicircular canal.

32 a) **True** About 93% of oral cavity lesions are benign. Of the malignant lesions, 90% are squamous cell cancers. Other malignancies include adenocarcinoma, adenoid cystic carcinoma, mucoepidermoid carcinoma, lymphoma and sarcoma.

b) **True** Pleomorphic adenomas are well-defined lesions with little contrast enhancement on CT. On MRI, they are isointense to muscle on T1-weighted scans and hyperintense on T2-weighted scans. They may have cystic, haemorrhagic or calcified areas.

c) **True** Spread occurs to the submandibular and internal jugular lymph node chain. This is usually bilateral.

d) **False** The most common sites of squamous cell carcinoma are the lower lip, oral tongue and floor of the mouth.

e) **False** Ranulas are mucous retention cysts of the floor of the mouth. They are simple unilocular cystic lesions. Rarely, they may dissect across the midline and present as bilateral masses.

33 a) **True** About 10%–20% occur in the parotid gland and 1%–7% in the sublingual gland.

b) **True**

c) **True** About 80% of submandibular stones and 60% of parotid stones are radio-opaque.

d) **True** About 85% of submandibular stones occur within Wharton's duct.

e) **True**

34 a) **False** The most common site of obstruction is at the junction of the lacrimal sac and nasolacrimal duct.

   b) **True**

   c) **True** Diverticula may resolve once the obstruction is removed.

   d) **True** Fistulae may be congenital, postinfectious, inflammatory or traumatic. They most commonly involve the lacrimal sac.

   e) **True** Normal DSG is always associated with normal contrast DCG. However, in 26% of cases in which DCG indicates a normal lacrimal system, DSG shows evidence of obstruction.

35 a) **True** Chordomas in the clivus may also involve the spheno-occipital synchondrosis. A total of 50% arise in the sacrum and 35% arise in the skull base. Metastasis, usually to the lungs, occurs in 7%.

   b) **True** Most show homogenous enhancement and speckled calcification.

   c) **True** Meningiomas may extend below the base of skull and rapidly enlarge. Most are uniformly enhancing lesions.

   d) **True** This is particularly true of petro-occipital synchondrosis, which, unlike chordomas, is not midline.

   e) **False** Local spread of tumour is the most frequent mode of proliferation. Other pathways include haematogenous and perineural spread.

36 a) **True** Due to its multiplanar capabilities and ability to visualise nerves and vessels, MRI is the preferred mode of investigation.

   b) **True** Trauma to the brachial plexus can result in avulsion of the nerve root and pseudomeningocoele. Distal trauma may cause neural oedema and haematoma and lead to posttraumatic neuroma.

   c) **True** Postradiotherapy brachial plexopathy typically presents within 1 year as weakness and lymphoedema.

   d) **True** On MRI, postradiotherapy fibrosis (with doses greater than 60 Gy) is often isointense to muscle on T1- and T2-weighted sequences. Tumour recurrence shows high signal on T2-weighted imaging and enhances with contrast.

   e) **True** However, myelography fails to demonstrate intradural rootlets at the involved level.

37 a) **True** Non-Hodgkin's disease more frequently involves Waldeyer's ring.

   b) **True** About 60% of non-Hodgkin's lymphomas involve extranodal sites, whereas 98% of patients with Hodgkin's disease have involvement of the nodes.

   c) **False** There is frequently no central necrosis.

   d) **False** Calcification is rarely described before treatment, but is common after chemoradiotherapy.

   e) **False** Orbital lymphoma is usually non-Hodgkin's lymphoma and more commonly involves the lacrimal gland and other extraconal structures than the intraconal elements. It may be bilateral.

38 a) **False** This is a localised tumour of immature myeloid cells. The mean age
at presentation is 48 years.

   b) **True** About 85% are solitary lesions.

   c) **True** Acute myeloid leukaemia, chronic myeloid leukaemia, polycythaemia rubra vera
and other myeloproliferative disorders may be associated in 48% of cases.

   d) **True** MRI shows intermediate signal on most sequences. Radiographs may show
poorly defined lytic bone lesions.

   e) **False** Head and neck lesions may involve the skull, face, orbits, paranasal sinuses
and nasal cavity.

39 a) **True** The motor fibres travel separately from the sensory fibres. Lesions affecting
the facial nerve within the cerebellopontine angle or the internal acoustic canal
also tend to affect the VIII cranial nerve.

   b) **True** The VII nerve courses beneath the lateral semicircular canal and above the oval
window. Dehiscence of the tegmen tympani allows the nerve to protrude into
the oval window, making it vulnerable during surgery.

   c) **False** Hemifacial spasm occurs in women and begins with tonic and clonic contraction
of facial muscles. The most common aetiology is a tortuous anterior inferior
cerebellar artery or posterior inferior cerebellar artery.

   d) **True** Schwannomas may affect the nerve at any point. They grow eccentrically.
Intense enhancement is seen with gadolinium on MRI.

   e) **False** There can be mild enhancement in normal individuals due to the accompanying
vessels. Intense enhancement suggests palsy or tumour.

40 a) **True**

   b) **True** It also contains the carotid artery, jugular vessels, cranial nerves (IX–XII)
and sympathetic chain.

   c) **True**

   d) **True** However, this is not useful in a mass with a short axis of less than 2 cm.

   e) **False** The most common pathology is lymphadenopathy, which may be metastatic,
lymphomatous or granulomatous.

Chapter 8

Paediatric radiology

1   **Regarding intussusception, which of the following are true?**
    a) The peak incidence is between 6 months and 2 years of age
    b) The majority of cases are ileoileal
    c) Ultrasound has a low sensitivity in diagnosis
    d) Pneumatic reduction has a lower perforation rate compared with hydrostatic reduction
    e) The risk of recurrence following a successful reduction is approximately 30%

2   **Which of the following fractures in a child are highly specific for nonaccidental injury?**
    a) Sternal fracture
    b) Vertebral spinous process fracture
    c) Posterior rib fractures
    d) Humeral shaft fracture
    e) Tibial shaft fracture

3   **Regarding hypertrophic pyloric stenosis, which of the following are true?**
    a) The peak incidence is between 2 and 6 months of age
    b) It is frequently diagnosed in premature infants
    c) Males and females are equally affected
    d) It is associated with gastric pneumatosis
    e) An elongated pyloric canal measuring 14 mm on ultrasound supports the diagnosis

4   **Regarding Meckel's diverticulum, which of the following are true?**
    a) It is a remnant of the omphalomesenteric duct
    b) It arises from the mesenteric border of the small bowel
    c) It is the most common identifiable cause of intussusception in children
    d) It is only diagnosed at angiography if there is active bleeding
    e) About 80%–90% contain ectopic gastric mucosa

5   **Regarding infantile polycystic kidney disease, which of the following are true?**
    a) It is inherited as an autosomal dominant condition
    b) The most common age of presentation is between 2 and 5 years of age
    c) Severe infantile polycystic disease is associated with severe hepatic fibrosis
    d) It typically reveals a striated nephrogram on the delayed excretory urogram
    e) Infantile polycystic kidneys are echopoor on ultrasound

6   **Which of the following statements are true?**
    a) Infratentorial tumours are more common than supratentorial tumours in the 2–5 years age group
    b) Medulloblastomas are the most common posterior fossa tumour in childhood
    c) Medulloblastomas are typically cystic lesions with a mural nodule
    d) Childhood brainstem gliomas predominantly arise in the midbrain
    e) Brainstem gliomas are prevalent in neurofibromatosis type I (NF-1)

7   **Regarding nonaccidental injuries, which of the following are true?**
    a) Shaken baby syndrome is typically seen between 1 year and 18 months of age
    b) Retinal haemorrhages are present in the majority of cases where shaking is involved
    c) Interhemispheric subdural haematomas are strongly associated with nonaccidental injury
    d) Extradural haematomas are highly suspicious of nonaccidental injury
    e) The 'white cerebellum sign' refers to posterior fossa haemorrhage following severe abuse

8 Regarding umbilical catheters, which of the following are true?
a) An umbilical venous catheter can be recognised by its caudal course from the umbilicus
b) The tip of an umbilical vein catheter may enter the pulmonary veins
c) The tip of an umbilical artery catheter should be positioned above T6
d) The normal umbilicus contains two veins and one artery
e) A common site of malposition of an umbilical vein catheter is with the tip in the middle hepatic vein

9 Regarding cleidocranial dysplasia, which of the following are true?
a) It is due to a sporadic genetic mutation
b) There is early closure of the cranial sutures
c) It is associated with mental retardation
d) Most patients are delivered by Caesarean section
e) Typically, patients have short second metacarpals

10 Causes of basal ganglia calcification in children include which of the following?
a) Down's syndrome
b) Wilson's disease
c) Cytomegalovirus infection
d) Hypoparathyroidism
e) Congenital rubella

11 Regarding developmental dysplasia of the hip, which of the following are true?
a) A prolonged labour is a recognised risk factor
b) The condition can be diagnosed on ultrasonography up to 18 months of age
c) Subluxation of 6–7 mm during ultrasound stress views of the hip is significant
d) Ultrasonographic examination is performed with the hip in a flexed position
e) The acetabular labrum is poorly seen on ultrasonography

12 Regarding retinoblastoma, which of the following are true?
a) Up to 40% of cases are inherited in an autosomal dominant fashion
b) Presentation is usually after 5 years of age
c) Tumour spread is typically along the optic nerve
d) A calcified intraocular mass is a characteristic computed tomography (CT) finding
e) There is an association with the later development of chondrosarcoma

13 In childhood, which of the following are true regarding non-Hodgkin's lymphoma?
a) Non-Hodgkin's lymphoma is more common than Hodgkin's disease in young children
b) Splenic involvement occurs in more than 70% of cases at presentation
c) There is a higher incidence of extranodal disease in childhood non-Hodgkin's lymphoma than when it occurs in adults
d) Pulmonary involvement is more common in Hodgkin's disease
e) Central nervous system disease at presentation indicates a poor prognosis

14 Regarding osteogenesis imperfecta, which of the following are true?
a) It results in intrauterine death in the majority of cases
b) It is associated with abnormally sclerotic bone
c) It is characteristically associated with wormian bones
d) Deafness is secondary to otosclerosis
e) It heals with a florid periosteal reaction around fractures

15 **Increased reflectivity is a prominent feature of ultrasonography of the infant brain in which of the following?**
   a) Interhemispheric lipoma
   b) Septo-optic dysplasia
   c) Cytomegalovirus infection
   d) Nonaccidental injury
   e) Periventricular leucomalacia

16 **Which of the following statements are true?**
   a) The maximum diameter of the normal appendix on ultrasonography should not be greater than 8 mm
   b) Increased echogenicity of the submucosal layer is a feature of perforation of the appendix
   c) In patients with appendiceal perforation, the appendix is visualised on ultrasonography in 80%–90% of cases
   d) Air within the appendix on CT is suspicious for appendicitis
   e) The presence of an appendicolith on ultrasonography or CT warrants an appendicectomy

17 **Regarding choanal atresia, which of the following are true?**
   a) It is usually due to membranous obstruction of the choanae
   b) Urgent treatment is required if the condition is bilateral
   c) Magnetic resonance imaging (MRI) is the modality of choice for diagnosis
   d) It is associated with cleft face, nose and palate
   e) The vomer is typically thickened on CT

18 **Regarding Arnold–Chiari type II malformation, which of the following are true?**
   a) It is characterised by dysgenesis of the cerebellar vermis
   b) There is hypoplasia of the cerebellum
   c) Spina bifida is strongly associated
   d) The spinal cord is frequently tethered
   e) It is associated with Klippel–Feil syndrome

19 **Regarding Wilms' tumour (nephroblastoma), which of the following are true?**
   a) Haematuria is a frequent presentation
   b) Calcification occurs less frequently than in neuroblastomas
   c) Lung metastases are common
   d) There is an association with NF
   e) The prognosis is poor

20 **Which of the following statements are true?**
   a) The normal thymus in a child is hypoechoic relative to the liver
   b) The thymus is highly vascular on colour Doppler ultrasonography
   c) The thymus arises from the third and fourth branchial pouches
   d) Thymolipomas are common causes of thymic enlargement in childhood
   e) Teratomas comprise the most common anterior mediastinal mass in childhood

21 Regarding the neonatal spine, which of the following are true?
a) The tip of the conus medullaris is located at L3 in healthy neonates
b) Diasatematomyelia typically occurs in the mid-thoracic region
c) Diasatematomyelia is associated with cord tethering
d) Lateral meningocoeles are associated with Marfan's syndrome
e) Spinal ultrasonography is indicated in babies with a subcutaneous lipoma overlying the spine

22 Causes of neonatal cholestasis include which of the following?
a) Septo-optic dysplasia
b) Alagille syndrome
c) Hypothyroidism
d) Cystic fibrosis
e) Maternal warfarin ingestion

23 Regarding congenital lobar emphysema, which of the following are true?
a) CT demonstrates multiple small cysts in the affected lung
b) It may present with complete opacification of the affected lobe
c) The left upper lobe is most frequently affected
d) It is associated with congenital heart disease
e) Insertion of a chest drain is often curative

24 Regarding cystic fibrosis, which of the following are true?
a) Pleural fluid is usually the first manifestation of pulmonary disease
b) Stenotic pancreatic duct segments are common
c) Lobar pneumonia predominantly affects the lower lobes
d) The abnormal gene is on the long arm of chromosome 7
e) The paranasal sinuses are radiographically opaque in almost all patients over 2 years of age

25 Which of the following statements are true?
a) The 'H' type tracheo-oesophageal fistula is the most common
b) Duplication cysts of the gastrointestinal tract are most common in the ileal region
c) Duodenal atresia usually presents with bilious vomiting
d) Duodenal duplication cysts are located on the convex border of the duodenum
e) Duodenal atresia is associated with malrotation of the small bowel

26 Which of the following statements are true?
a) A left-sided superior vena cava usually drains into the left atrium, resulting in a right-to-left shunt
b) Total anomalous pulmonary circulation is always associated with an atrial septal defect or patent foramen ovale
c) Partial anomalous pulmonary circulation is associated with a hypogenetic right lung
d) Bronchopulmonary sequestration characteristically occurs in the right paravertebral gutter
e) Cystic adenomatoid malformation (CAM) occurs with equal frequency in both lungs

27 **Which of the following statements are true?**
   a) Vesico-ureteric reflux usually occurs into the lower pole moiety of a complete ureteral duplication
   b) Ectopic ureterocoeles in duplex kidneys are more common in boys than girls
   c) Ectopic ureteral insertion in boys is always suprasphincteric
   d) An ectopic ureteral insertion may present with daytime incontinence in a girl
   e) Horseshoe kidneys are associated with a higher incidence of duplicated kidneys

28 **Which of the following statements are true?**
   a) Giant cell tumours of bone are most commonly seen in the 5–15 years age group
   b) Ewing's tumour rarely arises within flat bones
   c) Parosteal osteosarcomas have a peak in the 10–20 years age group
   d) Eosinophilic granuloma usually involves one bone only
   e) Ewing's tumours often demonstrate calcification on CT

29 **Which of the following statements are correct?**
   a) The gallbladder is implicated in approximately 20% of patients with biliary atresia
   b) Neonatal hepatitis cannot be distinguished from biliary atresia on ultrasonography
   c) The presence of radioisotope within the gastrointestinal tract following a hepato-iminodiacetic acid (HIDA) scan excludes biliary atresia
   d) Surgical repair of biliary atresia is best delayed until after 3 months of age
   e) Biliary atresia is associated with asplenia

30 **Causes of delayed bone age include which of the following?**
   a) Inflammatory bowel disease
   b) Turner's syndrome
   c) Obesity
   d) Pseudohypoparathyroidism
   e) Cleidocranial dysplasia

31 **Which of the following are true regarding slipped femoral capital epiphysis?**
   a) It represents a Salter–Harris type V injury
   b) It is bilateral in 20% of cases
   c) There is slight widening of the joint space
   d) The slip is typically in a posteromedial direction
   e) Ultrasonography is useful in confirming the diagnosis

32 **Regarding hepatoblastomas, which of the following are true?**
   a) Presentation is usually after 4 years of age
   b) Alpha-fetoprotein levels are not elevated
   c) Following intravenous contrast-enhanced CT, hepatoblastomas are hypodense relative to the surrounding liver
   d) Calcification is rarely seen
   e) MRI characteristics of hepatocellular carcinomas and hepatoblastomas are similar

33 Features of Wolman's disease include which of the following?
a) Nephrocalcinosis
b) Splenomegaly
c) An autosomal recessive mode of inheritance
d) Death between 20 and 30 years of age
e) Generalised osteosclerosis

34 Regarding necrotising enterocolitis, which of the following are true?
a) Presentation is usually seen in premature infants within 48 hours of birth
b) It usually involves the proximal small bowel
c) Portal vein gas demands urgent surgical intervention
d) There is a decreased incidence in neonates receiving enteral nutrition
e) Gastric dilatation is a radiographic finding

35 Features of rickets include which of the following?
a) A sclerotic rim around the epiphysis
b) A metaphyseal spur projecting at right angles to the long axis of the bone
c) 'Ground glass' osteoporosis
d) Craniotabes
e) Biconcave vertebral bodies

36 Regarding eosinophilic granuloma, which of the following are true?
a) Bone lesions are usually solitary
b) Vertebral pedicles are typically affected
c) The cranial vault is rarely involved
d) The mandible is rarely involved
e) A periosteal reaction is not seen on plain film

37 Regarding AIDS in children, which of the following are true?
a) *Pneumocystis carinii* pneumonia is uncommon in children
b) Kaposi's sarcoma is rarely seen
c) The incubation period is shorter than in adults
d) Hypoechoic areas are present in the neonatal basal ganglia
e) Lymphocytic interstitial pneumonitis is common

38 Causes of ascites in the neonate include which of the following?
a) Hydrops fetalis
b) Posterior urethral valves
c) Meconium peritonitis
d) Biliary atresia
e) Lymphangiectasia

39 Regarding wormian bones, which of the following are true?
a) They are a normal finding up to 18 months of age
b) They typically involve the coronal suture
c) They are a feature of Down's syndrome
d) They are seen in sickle cell anaemia
e) They are a feature of rickets

40 Regarding the paediatric parotid gland, which of the following are true?
  a) The normal parotid gland is hypoechoic relative to adjacent muscle
  b) An accessory parotid gland is present in 20% of patients
  c) The facial nerve is not visualised on any imaging modality
  d) Pleomorphic adenomas are extremely rare in the paediatric population
  e) Fluid–fluid interfaces are typical of haemangiomas on MRI

Answers

1 a) **True**   Approximately 50% of cases present in the first year of life and 24% in the second year. Two thirds are male.

   b) **False** More than 90% of cases are ileocolic. Only 4% are ileoileal.

   c) **False** Ultrasound is highly sensitive (90%–100%). Typically, a 'target' sign is seen on transverse imaging with a central hyperechoic area representing the mesentery of the intussusceptum and a surrounding hypoechoic ring representing the wall of the intussuscipiens.

   d) **False** Perforation rates are similar. Pneumatic methods are faster, however, allowing a lower radiation dose. There is also less peritoneal contamination in the event of a colonic perforation.

   e) **False** In the absence of a lead point (94% of cases in children are idiopathic), bowel wall oedema due to reduction of the intussusception tends to prevent any early recurrence.

2 a) **True**

   b) **True**

   c) **True**

   d) **True**   Metaphyseal 'corner' fractures are almost pathognomonic for nonaccidental injury. Sternal, scapular, humeral shaft, vertebral spinous process and posterior rib fractures are not normally seen in children and, therefore, also have a high specificity for nonaccidental injury. Fractures of different ages, irrespective of the site of injury, or fractures through previous callus formation should also raise strong suspicions.

   e) **False** Spiral tibial shaft fractures in children are common injuries, often as a result of a rotational force applied during a fall. An incomplete, oblique hairline crack in the distal tibia sustained when the child is learning to walk is termed a 'toddler's fracture'.

3 a) **False** There is a peak incidence between 2 and 6 weeks of age.

   b) **False** For reasons that are unclear, it is an extremely rare diagnosis in premature infants.

   c) **False** It typically occurs in firstborn males (M:F = 4:1) with an incidence of 1:1000. It results from hypertrophy of the circular muscle fibres of the pylorus. The aetiology is unknown.

   d) **True**   Gastric pneumatosis is occasionally identified on plain abdominal X-ray. Following decompression of the stomach, the pneumatosis rapidly resolves. Other associations include: oesophageal atresia, tracheo-oesophageal fistula, hiatal hernia, Turner's syndrome, trisomy 18 and congenital rubella.

   e) **False** The pyloric canal length should measure at least 17 mm, the pyloric wall thickness at least 3 mm and the transverse diameter of the pylorus at least 13 mm in order to make the diagnosis on ultrasound.

4 a) **True** This is also known as the vitelline duct and connects the midgut to the yolk sac in the embryo. It is seen in 2% of the population, measures 5 cm in length, lies within 60 cm of the terminal ileum and, if symptomatic, usually presents before 2 years of age.

b) **False** They are true diverticula, containing all four intestinal wall layers. They arise from the antimesenteric border of the bowel.

c) **True** The vast majority of intussusceptions in children are of unknown cause. Meckel's diverticulum is the most common lead point identified. Other causes include polyps, enteric and duplication cysts, and Henoch–Schönlein purpura.

d) **False** A long, nonbranching ileal artery typically supplies Meckel's diverticulum. This may be an incidental finding at angiography.

e) **False** Only 50% contain ectopic gastric mucosa. These can be detected using technetium-99m-labelled pertechnetate.

5 a) **False** Adult-type polycystic kidney disease shows autosomal dominant inheritance with gene defects identified on chromosomes 16 and 4. Infantile polycystic kidney disease is inherited in an autosomal recessive fashion.

b) **False** The most common type is the antenatal form. This condition presents *in utero* and progresses to renal failure and pulmonary hypoplasia (Potter sequence), with the majority of patients dying in the first 24 hours of life.

c) **False** The milder forms (neonatal, infantile and juvenile types) present in the first few years of life and are associated with more severe hepatic fibrosis: the less severe the renal disease, the more severe the hepatic abnormalities.

d) **True** This appearance is caused by stasis of contrast material in dilated tubules. The kidneys are symmetrically enlarged and have a smooth outline.

e) **False** The affected kidneys are replaced by a multitude of small elongated cysts representing dilated tubules and collecting ducts. These cysts are too small to delineate on ultrasound, but produce an echogenic pattern due to multiple interfaces of the walls of the dilated ducts. There is poor corticomedullary differentiation.

6 a) **True** Infratentorial neoplasms predominate in the 2–5 years age group. Supratentorial tumours become more common in the second decade of life.

b) **True** Medulloblastomas comprise 30%–40% of all posterior fossa neoplasms in childhood. Cerebellar astrocytomas are the second most common.

c) **False** This typically describes a cerebellar astrocytoma. Medulloblastomas are typically densely cellular midline tumours. Both tumour types may obstruct the fourth ventricle.

d) **False** About 40%–60% of brainstem gliomas arise in the pons, with only 15%–20% occurring in the midbrain.

e) **True** T2-weighted high signal within the brainstem with associated mass effect and cranial nerve involvement is typical of a brainstem glioma in a child with NF type I.

7 a) **False** The average age of presentation is 6 months. Older children have a greater ability to withstand the effects of sudden acceleration and deceleration when shaken.

   b) **True** Beyond the neonatal period, when retinal haemorrhages are commonly seen as a consequence of the delivery, retinal haemorrhages are a highly specific sign of nonaccidental and intracranial injury.

   c) **True** These collections are often in the posterior interhemispheric fissure and are associated with violent shaking of the baby's head. Convexity subdural haematomas are usually also present, although they may only be seen on MRI.

   d) **False** Extradural haematomas are infrequent in infancy and are rarely seen in cases of abuse.

   e) **False** Severely injured infants may develop marked brain oedema secondary to ischaemia and hypoxia. This predominantly affects the cerebral cortex and deep white matter tracts and spares the basal ganglia and cerebellum. The relatively high density of the basal ganglia has been termed the reversal sign and the increased cerebellar density the 'white cerebellum sign'.

8 a) **False** The umbilical vein catheter enters the umbilical vein, ascends into the left portal vein to the ductus venosus and into the inferior vena cava and the right atrium.

   b) **True** The catheter tip may be advanced through the patent foramen ovale, into the left atrium and into a pulmonary vein. If the catheter crosses the midline, this should be suspected and the catheter should be withdrawn into the right atrium.

   c) **False** The umbilical artery catheter passes caudal from the umbilicus with a sharp bend near the superior margin of the sacroiliac joint as the catheter passes from the umbilical artery into the internal iliac artery and into the aorta. The catheter tip should lie between T6 and L4.

   d) **False** It contains two arteries and one vein.

   e) **True** An abrupt reversal of direction of the umbilical vein catheter below the diaphragm often implies that the catheter has entered the middle hepatic vein.

9 a) **False** It is transmitted as an autosomal dominant condition.

   b) **False** There is widening of the cranial sutures/fontanelles with delayed closure. There is often a persistent metopic suture.

   c) **False**

   d) **True** Patients usually have a large head, resulting in the need for delivery by Caesarean section.

   e) **False** The second metacarpals are often elongated. Other features of the hand include pointed terminal tufts, coned epiphyses and squared-off metacarpal bases. Hypoplastic clavicles, delayed dentition, wormian bones and extra ribs are the other classical features.

10 All true The cause of basal ganglia calcification is unclear in the majority of cases and has no clinical significance. The basal ganglia are susceptible to insults early in life due to their high energy requirements. There are multiple other causes of calcification, including birth anoxia, hypoparathyroidism, pseudohypoparathyroidism, pseudopseudohypoparathyroidism, hyperparathyroidism, AIDS, tuberculosis, toxoplasmosis, cysticercosis, poisoning (e.g. lead, carbon monoxide), chemotherapy, radiotherapy, Fahr's disease, Cockayne's syndrome and childhood infections. Wilson's disease causes low attenuation lesions in the basal ganglia on CT, but can also cause calcification.

11 a) False A breech delivery, family history, female sex, oligohydramnios and neuromuscular disorders are all risk factors for developmental dysplasia.

  b) **False** Ossification of the femoral head limits the use of ultrasound beyond 8–10 months.

  c) **True** Up to 5 mm of subluxation can be within normal limits. Beyond this indicates significant instability. The influence of maternal hormones causes subluxation of up to 6 mm in neonates; therefore, the study should not be performed until the baby is more than 2 weeks of age.

  d) **True** Both the neutral and stressed views are performed with the hip in the flexed position. The stressed manoeuvre is a posterior push with the hip flexed and adducted.

  e) **False** The labrum is well demonstrated. The lateral tip and juxta-osseous portions are echogenic, whilst the mid portion is echopoor.

12 a) True The genetic abnormality has been localised to chromosome 13. The majority of cases are due to a sporadic gene mutation.

  b) **False** Most cases (98%) occur before 5 years of age. A total of 30% of tumours are bilateral and 30% are multifocal within one eye. Trilateral retinoblastoma refers to the rare variant of bilateral retinoblastoma and neuroectodermal pineal tumour (pineoblastoma).

  c) **True** Metastases typically occur along the optic nerve via the subarachnoid space. Metastases also commonly occur in meninges, bone marrow, lung, liver and lymph nodes.

  d) **True** CT reveals a lobulated, dense mass that shows some degree of calcification in up to 95% of cases. In the absence of calcifications, other mass lesions should be suspected, such as persistent primary hyperplastic vitreous, retrolental fibroplasia, toxocariasis, and Coats' disease.

  e) **True** Patients with the inherited form of retinoblastoma are at increased risk of other nonocular tumours, of which osteosarcoma is the most common. Other nonocular tumours include chondrosarcoma, fibrosarcoma and malignant fibrous histiocytoma.

13 a) **True** It is also three times more common in boys. Immunodeficiency syndromes increase the risk of non-Hodgkin's lymphoma.

  b) **False** Abdominal involvement usually presents with a mass, typically in the ileocaecal region, or intussusception causing obstruction. Splenic involvement is present in less than 40% of cases at presentation.

  c) **True** Childhood non-Hodgkin's lymphoma also tends to be of a higher histological grade, with a diffuse pattern being more common than a follicular pattern.

  d) **True** Pulmonary involvement is twice as common in Hodgkin's disease as in non-Hodgkin's lymphoma.

  e) **True** Any central nervous system involvement is considered as stage IV disease.

14 a) **False** Four types of osteogenesis imperfecta are classically described. Type I is the most common and is compatible with life. Type II is usually fatal in the neonatal period, with 50% being stillborn. Type III and IV are rare.

  b) **False** There is diffuse osteopenia with a reduced trabecular pattern.

  c) **True** Other changes in the skull include: marked thinning of the calvarium, platybasia, mastoid cell enlargement and otosclerosis.

  d) **True** This is typically seen in type I osteogenesis imperfecta secondary to a thickened, undermineralised otic capsule.

  e) **True** Exuberant callus formation may be seen around fracture sites.

15 a) **True**

  b) **False** This condition is characterised by hypoplasia of the optic nerves and hypoplasia of the septum pellucidum.

  c) **True** Other central nervous system manifestations of cytomegalovirus infection include periventricular calcification, ventricular dilatation and microcephaly.

  d) **True** This is usually due to subdural blood, which is often in the interhemispheric region.

  e) **True** This represents necrosis of deep white matter tracts secondary to ischaemia, and is seen in premature infants. Typically, there is periventricular echogenicity, which becomes apparent 2 days to 2 weeks following an ischaemic insult. With time, periventricular cystic change occurs.

16 a) **False** The upper limit of normal is 6 mm. The inflamed appendix is typically a fluid filled, noncompressible, blind-ending, tubular structure.

  b) **False** An echogenic submucosal layer is typically seen in an inflamed, but not perforated, appendix.

  c) **False** The appendix is visible in only 40%–60% of patients with appendiceal perforation. Secondary features of perforation include the presence of a loculated periappendicular or pelvic fluid collection or abscess.

  d) **False** Thin collimation CT often shows air within the normal appendix.

  e) **True** This is true even in asymptomatic patients. About 50% of patients will have a perforation or abscess at surgery.

17 a) **False** More than 90% of cases are due to an osseous obstruction. Choanal atresia results from failed perforation of the oronasal membrane.

b) **True** Neonates are obligate nose breathers in the first 2–6 months of life. Bilateral choanal atresia, therefore, causes respiratory distress that is only relieved by crying. Immediate measures are required to secure an airway.

c) **False** CT scanning with the patient prone and the gantry angled 5°–10° cephalad to the hard palate is the imaging modality of choice.

d) **True** There are several associated conditions, including amniotic band syndrome, malrotation of the bowel, DiGeorge syndrome, Treacher Collins' syndrome and craniosynostosis. Overall, 50% of cases of choanal atresia are associated with other anomalies.

e) **True** The main CT imaging features are narrowing of the posterior choanae to less than 0.34 cm in children aged under 2 years, inward bowing of the posterior maxilla, thickening of the vomer and the presence of a bone or soft-tissue septum across the posterior choanae.

18 a) **False** This is present in the Dandy–Walker malformation.

b) **False** This is typical of the Chiari IV malformation.

c) **True** Chiari II malformation is the most common Chiari malformation and is the result of a small posterior fossa with resultant downward displacement of the cerebellum, fourth ventricle and brain stem. There is herniation of the cerebellar vermis and tonsils through the foramen magnum and a lumbar myelomeningocoele is almost always present.

d) **True** This has been suggested as the underlying aetiology of the condition.

e) **False** This is present in 10% of Chiari I malformations.

19 a) **False** Wilms' tumour typically presents as an abdominal mass in a healthy child. Other presentations include hypertension and abdominal pain. Fever and haematuria are rare.

b) **True** Calcification is seen in 90% of neuroblastomas, but in only 10% of Wilms' tumours.

c) **True** Neuroblastoma tends to metastasise to bone.

d) **False** There is an association with aniridia, hemihypertrophy and urogenital disorders (horseshoe kidney, cryptorchidism and hypospadia).

e) **False** Long-term survival is achieved in 90% of patients. This is mainly due to oncological advances.

20 a) **True** The gland has a granular echotexture with echogenic strands. It has a smooth, well-defined margin.

b) **False** The normal thymus is hypovascular.

c) **True** This explains the occasional presence of thymic tissue in the neck.

d) **False** Thymomas and thymolipomas are extremely rare in childhood. Neoplastic involvement is usually secondary to infiltration by leukaemia or lymphoma.

e) **False** Thymic hyperplasia is the most common cause. This may be secondary to hyperthyroidism, myasthenia gravis and rebound growth following illness or stress.

21 a) **False** The tip is located at L1/L2 and should never be present below L3.

b) **False** Diastematomyelia is most commonly seen at the thoraco-lumbar junction. There is a sagittal cleft in the spinal cord with either a fibrous, cartilaginous or osseous septum. Ultrasonography will demonstrate both hemicords in cross-section, although presence of a bony septum may prevent good visualisation.

c) **True** About 50% of patients will have cord tethering. Spinal ultrasonography may also demonstrate associated hydromyelia, syringomyelia and a thickened filum terminale.

d) **True** Lateral meningoceles are cerebrospinal fluid (CSF)-filled protrusions of dura and arachnoid mater through an enlarged intervertebral foramen. They are associated with Marfan's syndrome, Ehlers–Danlos syndrome and NF.

e) **True** Any cutaneous lesion overlying the spine may be a marker of underlying spinal pathology. Further indications include spinal scoliosis, sacral malformations, bladder or bowel dysfunction and suspected spinal injury secondary to birth trauma.

22 a) **True** This is a mild form of lobar holoprosencephaly that is associated with neonatal cholestasis. It is characterised by absence of the septum pellucidum, squared frontal horns of the lateral ventricles and hypoplasia of the optic nerve and chiasm.

b) **True** There is paucity and hypoplasia of the intrahepatic bile ducts. Affected patients have abnormal facies, vertebral arch defects and congenital heart disease. The condition is progressive.

c) **True**

d) **True** Plugging of the biliary tract causes obstruction in the neonate. Other inherited causes of neonatal cholestasis include α1-antitrypsin deficiency, galactosaemia and hereditary tyrosinaemia.

e) **False** This is associated with skeletal and neurological anomalies.

23 a) **False** Congenital lobar emphysema represents an over-inflated lobe that compresses the normal adjacent lung. Cysts are not a feature. About 50% of cases are idiopathic and the rest are caused by an airway obstruction (e.g. bronchial cartilage deficiency, mucus, web, stenosis or extrinsic compression).

b) **True** Foetal lung fluid becomes trapped within the lobe, resulting in an opaque, expanded lobe. This converts to the typical hyperlucent lobe once the fluid has drained or been absorbed.

c) **True** The left upper lobe is affected in 40% of cases, the right middle lobe in 35% of cases and the right upper lobe in 20%. Two lobes are affected in only 5% of cases.

d) **True** In 15% of cases, there is a patent ductus arteriosus or ventriculoseptal defect.

e) **False** In most cases, treatment is expectant. Surgical excision is sometimes required.

24 a) **False** Pleural effusions are rare. Hyperinflation is usually the first radiological manifestation of lung disease.

b) **False** Progressive duct dilatation and ectasia with pancreatic atrophy are the typical features. This is due to obstruction by protein plugs.

c) **False** There is right upper lobe predominance. Poor mucous clearance encourages *Pseudomonas aeruginosa* infection.

d) **True** This gene codes for an abnormal chloride-ion transport protein.

e) **True** This is usually due to mucosal hypertrophy rather than active infection.

25 a) **False** The 'H' type tracheo-oesophageal fistula comprises only 10% of cases. Upper oesophageal atresia with a fistulous connection between the trachea and the lower oesophagus is the most common type (85%).

b) **True** Oesophageal duplications are the second most common.

c) **True** The obstruction is usually beyond the ampulla of Vater. Typically, vomiting is delayed until after the first feed. A 'double bubble' is seen on the plain abdominal X-ray.

d) **False** Duodenal duplication cysts are usually situated along the concave border where they may cause duodenal obstruction, biliary obstruction or pancreatitis.

e) **True** Associated anomalies occur in 50% of cases, including: malrotation of the small bowel, oesophageal atresia, congenital heart disease, imperforate anus, annular pancreas and Down's syndrome.

26 a) **False** An anomalous left-sided superior vena cava usually drains into the right atrium via the coronary sinus. Uncommonly, it drains into the left atrium causing a right-to-left shunt.

b) **True** In total anomalous pulmonary circulation, the total pulmonary venous return drains into the systemic venous circulation. A right-to-left shunt is required to maintain systemic circulation.

c) **True** This is termed the 'scimitar syndrome' due to the characteristic shape of the right pulmonary veins draining into the inferior vena cava.

d) **False** About 66% of intralobar sequestrations and 90% of extralobar sequestrations arise in the left lung base.

e) **True** CAM is slightly more frequent in the upper lobes. The differential diagnoses of CAM include diaphragmatic hernia, congenital lobar emphysema and lung sequestration.

27 a) **True** Vesico-ureteric reflux is the most common complication of complete ureteral duplication. It is more common in girls than boys and is due to the lower pole ureter having a more superolateral position as it enters the bladder and, therefore, a shorter intramural tunnel.

b) **False** Ureterocoeles, which are related to the upper pole moiety of a duplex kidney, occur eight times more frequently in girls than boys. Ureterocoeles related to a nonduplicated system show an equal gender incidence.

c) **True** The ureter arises from the wolffian ducts, which in males form the seminal vesicles, vas deferens, ejaculatory ducts and the prostatic urethra. These structures are proximal to the external sphincter so that ectopic ureteral insertion does not cause incontinence. In girls, wolffian duct remnants are present in the vagina, urethra and Gartner's ducts, which are beyond the sphincters, so that ectopic ureteral insertion results in incontinence.

d) **True** Incontinence may be present only during the day as the dilated ectopic ureter can act as a reservoir for urine whilst the patient is lying flat at night.

e) **True** There are associated anomalies in 50% of cases including ureteropelvic junction obstruction (seen in 30% of cases), ureteral duplication (10%), hypospadia, cryptorchidism, bicornuate uterus, trisomy 18 and Turner's syndrome.

28 a) **False** The majority of giant cell tumours occur in patients following fusion of the epiphyses. They have a narrow zone of transition and usually abut the articular margin.

  b) **False** About 60% arise in long bones, most commonly the metadiaphysis of the femur. About 40% arise in flat bones, particularly the pelvis. In patients over 20 years of age, the tumour predominantly arises in flat bones.

  c) **False** Parosteal osteosarcomas occur in an older age group than the periosteal type, with 50% occurring after 30 years of age.

  d) **True** The process is monostotic in 50%–75% of cases. The skull vault is most commonly involved.

  e) **False** Calcification is rare in Ewing's tumour of the bone. Ewing's typically presents with an 'onion skin' periosteal reaction on plain film.

29 a) **True** Although typically the gallbladder is not visualised in biliary atresia, a smaller than expected gallbladder is demonstrated in 20% of cases.

  b) **True** In 10% of cases of neonatal hepatitis, the gallbladder is not identified. Therefore, ultrasonography alone is not sufficient to distinguish these two conditions.

  c) **True** However, in severe forms of neonatal hepatitis, the liver may be sufficiently damaged to prevent enough radioisotope reaching the duodenum to be detected. The classical appearance of biliary atresia on an HIDA scan is good hepatic activity after 5 minutes, but no bowel visualisation after 24 hours.

  d) **False** If surgical repair (Kasai operation) is performed before 2 months of age, there is a 90% success rate. After 3 months, the success rate falls to under 20%.

  e) **False** Polysplenia is seen in 10%–15% of patients with biliary atresia.

30 a) **True**
  b) **True**
  c) **False**
  d) **False**
  e) **True**

Any systemic chronic illness can delay bone maturation. Metabolic causes include: hypopituitarism, hypothyroidism, hypogonadism, diabetes mellitus and rickets. Hypoparathyroidism accelerates maturation of bone, with early fusion of growth plates resulting in dwarfism. Obesity can also accelerate bone maturation.

31 a) **False** It is a slip of the epiphyseal plate, which is a Salter–Harris type I injury. A Salter–Harris type V injury describes a crush injury to the growth plate and is associated with growth impairment in almost 100% of cases. The prognosis in a type I injury is favourable.

b) **True** It is more common in overweight male teenagers. There is a history of trauma in 50% of cases.

c) **False** Joint space widening is seen in Perthes disease. In slipped femoral capital epiphysis, there is widening and irregularity of the epiphyseal plate.

d) **True** Hence the need for the 'frog-leg' view. The antero-posterior film is normal in 10% of cases.

e) **False** CT may demonstrate a decreased angle of femoral neck anteversion. Slipped capital femoral epiphysis may be complicated by avascular necrosis of the femoral head (15%), chondrolysis (10%), varus ('pistol-grip') deformity, degenerative osteoarthritis and limb-length discrepancy due to premature physeal closure.

32 a) **False** Hepatoblastomas typically present as an abdominal mass in an asymptomatic child aged under 2 years. Hepatocellular carcinomas present in children over 4 years of age.

b) **False** Both hepatoblastomas and hepatocellular carcinomas produce elevated alpha-fetoprotein levels. Hepatoblastomas are associated with hemihypertrophy and Beckwith–Wiedemann syndrome.

c) **True** Hepatoblastomas typically enhance to a lesser degree than the surrounding liver on CT imaging.

d) **False** Calcification is present on CT in 50% of cases.

e) **True** Both tumours are inhomogenous on MRI and return a lower T1 signal and higher T2 signal than the surrounding liver.

33 a) **False** There is typically bilateral punctate adrenal calcification. The adrenal glands are enlarged.

b) **True** Hepatosplenomegaly occurs due to deposition of cholesterol esters and triglycerides. Other imaging features include enlarged lymph nodes and small bowel wall thickening, both of which are due to fatty infiltration.

c) **True** The condition is due to a lack of lysosomal lipase/esterase.

d) **False** Death occurs within the first 6 months of life.

e) **False** Osteoporosis is a feature.

34 a) **False** The condition typically occurs more than 48 hours after birth, with very few cases developing beyond 2 weeks of life. As well as prematurity, another risk factor is bowel obstruction (e.g. Hirschsprung's disease, small bowel atresia, pyloric stenosis, meconium ileus and meconium plug syndrome).

b) **False** The terminal ileum followed by the caecum and ascending colon are most frequently involved.

c) **False** Although a serious finding, portal vein gas can be a transient appearance and on its own does not warrant urgent surgery.

d) **False** Approximately 90% of neonates with necrotising enterocolitis have received enteral nutrition.

e) **True** Other features include a persistently dilated bowel loop, an unchanging bowel gas pattern, pneumatosis intestinalis and portal vein gas.

35 a) **False** This is typical of scurvy (Wimberger's sign). The epiphysis in rickets is typically poorly mineralised and appears late.

   b) **True** The classical features of rickets are cupping and fraying of the metaphysis, with irregular widening of the epiphyseal plate.

   c) **False** Coarse trabeculations are seen in rickets. A ground glass appearance is characteristic of scurvy.

   d) **True** The poorly mineralised occiput becomes flattened in the supine baby. This is accentuated by frontal bossing.

   e) **True** Other imaging findings are bowing deformities of the long bones, delayed closure of the fontanelles, periosteal reaction and enlargement of costochondral junctions ('rachitic rosary').

36 a) **True** About 75% of cases are monostotic.

   b) **False** Eosinophilic granuloma typically involves the vertebral body, most commonly the thoracic spine, causing vertebra plana. It rarely involves the posterior elements and the disc spaces are preserved.

   c) **False** The skull is the most frequent site of involvement. Typically, there is a round or oval lucency within the skull vault with a bevelled edge.

   d) **False** It often involves the mandible, causing a 'floating teeth' appearance.

   e) **False** Although a periosteal reaction is almost never seen in flat bones, a prominent periosteal reaction is not unusual in the axial skeleton. This may simulate a neoplastic lesion.

37 a) **False** *P. carinii* pneumonia is the most common opportunistic infection in children. Hypoxia is usually severe. There is typically airspace shadowing, but unusual features, such as calcified hilar and mediastinal nodes, are not uncommon.

   b) **True**

   c) **True**

   d) **False** Nonspecific hyperechoic lesions are seen in the basal ganglia of neonatal HIV-seropositive patients. Other causes include cytomegalovirus, toxoplasmosis, rubella and asphyxia.

   e) **True** Lymphocytic interstitial pneumonitis is rare in adults but is the most common pulmonary complication of AIDS in children. A diffuse reticulonodular pattern is usually seen.

38 a) **True** The presence of ascites indicates severe anaemia.

   b) **True** Increasing back pressure results in extravasation of urine into the perirenal tissues and subsequently into the peritoneal cavity.

   c) **True** Meconium peritonitis typically causes linear calcifications over the serosal surfaces of the bowel and abdominal organs. This is due to *in utero* bowel perforation and is associated with air–fluid levels within the peritoneal cavity.

   d) **True** Presentation is typically with jaundice and hepatosplenomegaly. As cirrhosis progresses, ascites becomes a feature.

   e) **True** Blockage of the lymphatic system due to intestinal lymphangiectasia results in chylous ascites.

39 a) **False** They are a normal finding up to 6–12 months of age.
   b) **False** They typically involve the lambdoid and posterior sagittal sutures, extending around the posterior fontanelle.
   c) **True**
   d) **False** Sickle cell anaemia, as well as other types of anaemia, classically causes a 'hair-on-end' appearance in the cranial vault.
   e) **True** They are a feature during the healing phase. They are also seen in osteogenesis imperfecta, cleidocranial dysplasia, hypothyroidism, hypophosphatasia, pyknodysostosis, pachydermoperiostosis, progeria, kinky hair syndrome and as an idiopathic finding.

40 a) **False** The paediatric parotid gland is homogenous and hyperechoic relative to muscle.
   b) **True** An accessory parotid gland lies superficial to the masseter muscle and anterior to the main gland. It drains directly into the parotid duct.
   c) **False** MRI is consistently able to demonstrate the facial nerve. Ultrasonography and CT are not reliable in this regard.
   d) **False** Pleomorphic adenomas are the third most common tumour of the paediatric parotid gland after haemangiomas and lymphangiomas.
   e) **False** Fluid–fluid interfaces are typical of lymphangiomas. The appearance is due to haemorrhage within the cystic spaces.

Chapter 9

Breast imaging

---

1   **Which of the following are true regarding screening tests for breast cancer in the general population?**
    a) Screening mammography has been shown to reduce mortality from breast cancer
    b) Screening using ultrasound has been shown to reduce breast cancer mortality in patients less than 35 years old
    c) In the UK, mammographic screening is currently advocated for women aged over 40 years
    d) Cancers showing casting linear calcifications on mammography are associated with a poorer prognosis
    e) Two views of the breast are obtained for all screening assessments

2   **Which of the following are causes of a spiculated lesion on mammography?**
    a) Fat necrosis
    b) Medullary carcinoma
    c) Cystosarcoma phyllodes
    d) Postoperative haematoma
    e) Plasma cell mastitis

3   **Which of the following are true regarding noninvasive breast cancer?**
    a) Spotted calcifications on mammography are typical of high-grade ductal carcinoma *in situ* (DCIS)
    b) DCIS accounts for 20%–40% of nonpalpable cancers diagnosed on mammography
    c) The diagnosis of DCIS cannot be made using ultrasonography or magnetic resonance imaging (MRI)
    d) High-grade DCIS is associated with increased expression of the c-erb B-2 oncogene
    e) Lobular carcinoma *in situ* frequently presents as a mass lesion on mammography

4   **Which of the following are true regarding invasive breast cancers?**
    a) Rim calcification is frequently seen in medullary carcinoma
    b) There is an association between tubular carcinoma and radial scar
    c) Colloid carcinoma has a worse prognosis than invasive ductal carcinoma
    d) The most common invasive cancer in the male breast is invasive lobular carcinoma
    e) The likelihood of axillary spread of invasive ductal carcinoma depends on the size of the tumour

5   **Which of the following statements are true?**
    a) Radial scar is associated with a carcinoma in 30% of cases
    b) Plasma cell mastitis is typically unilateral and asymmetrical
    c) Lymphoma of the breast is more common in males
    d) Metastases to the breast most frequently present as a solitary mass
    e) A galactocoele appears radiolucent on mammography

6   **Which of the following ultrasonographic appearances of axillary lymph nodes are reportedly associated with malignant infiltration?**
    a) Rounded appearance of the lymph node
    b) Loss or displacement of the central fatty hilum
    c) An increase in vascular resistive index
    d) An increase in vascular pulsatility index
    e) Peripheral vascular flow pattern on colour or power Doppler imaging

7 **Which of the following are true of calcifications detected on mammography?**
   a) Skin calcifications typically have central lucent centres
   b) Milk of calcium has a typical appearance on the cranio-caudal view
   c) Sutural calcifications are usually linear in appearance
   d) Bilateral scattered punctate calcifications are probably benign
   e) Rim calcification is a feature of fat necrosis

8 **On MRI of silicone breast implants, which of the following are true?**
   a) Radial folds are secondary to infolding of the implant shell
   b) Radial folds appear thinner than lines associated with intracapsular rupture
   c) Extracapsular rupture is more common than intracapsular rupture
   d) The linguine sign is a feature of extracapsular rupture
   e) The keyhole sign describes the presence of a gel bleed

9 **Which of the following statements are true regarding fibroadenomas?**
   a) They are clinically palpable in the majority of cases
   b) They occur bilaterally in 25% of cases
   c) The incidence is higher in women receiving hormone replacement therapy
   d) They typically demonstrate posterior acoustic shadowing on ultrasonography
   e) Internal septations are typical on gadolinium-enhanced MRI

10 **Which of the following are true regarding breast cysts?**
   a) They are most frequently found in women aged under 30 years
   b) They are frequently multiple and bilateral
   c) They should be aspirated to exclude intracystic carcinoma
   d) They are prone to recurrent infection
   e) They may be indistinguishable from fibroadenomas on ultrasonography

11 **Which of the following are causes of posterior acoustic shadowing on breast ultrasonography?**
   a) DCIS
   b) Invasive ductal carcinoma
   c) Cooper's ligaments
   d) Ruptured silicone breast implant
   e) Surgical scar

12 **In the staging of invasive breast carcinoma, which of the following are true?**
   a) A tumour greater than 5 cm in size indicates T3 disease
   b) Involvement of internal mammary lymph nodes indicates N3 disease
   c) Ultrasound tends to overestimate the size of the primary tumour
   d) Mammography tends to underestimate the size of the primary tumour
   e) MRI is the most sensitive test in the detection of multifocal disease

13 **Which of the following statements are true?**
   a) Rheumatoid arthritis is associated with bilateral axillary lymphadenopathy
   b) There is an association between mastopathy and type 2 diabetes mellitus
   c) Fibromatosis is indistinguishable from an invasive carcinoma on mammography
   d) About 10% of cystosarcoma phyllodes cases result in distant metastases
   e) Metastases to the breast are frequently associated with overlying skin retraction

14 Which of the following are true regarding sclerosing adenosis?
   a) It commonly presents as focal or diffuse calcification
   b) It is a condition with high premalignant potential
   c) Biopsy is required to make a definitive diagnosis
   d) It presents with a palpable mass in the majority of cases
   e) It has an association with lobular carcinoma

15 Which of the following are true regarding fat necrosis of the breast?
   a) It is more common in asthenic women
   b) It tends to occur in a superficial or periareolar location
   c) Breast irradiation is a cause
   d) The presence of skin retraction makes fat necrosis unlikely
   e) Microcalcifications may occur

16 Which of the following are true regarding the mammographic changes following breast conserving surgery?
   a) Postoperative fluid collections should not persist for more than 3 months following surgery
   b) Parenchymal scarring typically contains areas of fat density
   c) New calcifications at 12 months following surgery are indicative of tumour recurrence
   d) Radiation treatment results in an increase in breast density
   e) Skin thickening should not persist for more than 3 months following radiation treatment

17 Which of the following are appropriate uses of ultrasonographic evaluation of the breasts?
   a) Differentiating solid from cystic lesions
   b) Evaluation of a palpable abnormality
   c) Evaluation of a suspected breast abscess
   d) Evaluation of a young woman with breast pain
   e) Evaluation of the asymptomatic, mammographically dense breast

18 Which of the following are true regarding breast biopsy?
   a) Core biopsy of a solid nodule is best performed using an 18G cutting needle
   b) In cases of suspicious microcalcifications, 10 or more core biopsies should be obtained
   c) Stereotactic needle biopsy involves generating a pair of mammographic images that are typically 5° off-centre on either side
   d) Specimen radiography is essential following biopsy for microcalcifications
   e) Mammotomy is most useful in the biopsy of microcalcifications

19 Which of the following are causes of a well-circumscribed lesion on mammography?
   a) Intramammary lymph node
   b) Intraductal papilloma
   c) Galactocoele
   d) Lipoma
   e) Breast haematoma

20 Which of the following statements are true regarding breast imaging?

   a) The presence of a halo sign on mammography is indicative of benignity
   b) MRI of the breast should ideally be avoided between days 6 and 16 of the menstrual cycle
   c) MRI is more sensitive than mammography in diagnosing Paget's disease of the nipple
   d) Early peripheral enhancement of a lesion on MRI is a feature of malignancy
   e) On MRI with intravenous gadolinium, malignant tumours typically demonstrate early rapid enhancement followed by washout of contrast

Answers

1   a) **True**   Screening mammography has been shown to reduce mortality from breast cancer by up to 32%. In the Swedish two-county trial, it was found that mammographic screening continued to save lives for up to 20 years. This is because screening improves the diagnosis of early cancers and is also able to identify subpopulations with a poorer prognosis that may benefit from more aggressive or adjuvant treatment.

    b) **False**   Ultrasonography currently has no role as a screening tool in any age group. However, targeted ultrasound is useful in patients with specific breast symptoms, clinically palpable abnormality or indeterminate mammographic abnormalities.

    c) **False**   Screening is currently available in the UK for patients who are 50–65 years old. Although the greatest benefits of screening appear in the 50–69 year age group, there is some evidence that screening also reduces mortality in the 40–49 year age group. This is currently being evaluated. There is also a plan to extend the UK's screening programme to include the 66–70 year age group.

    d) **True**   For small cancers (1–9 mm) detected by screening mammography, tumours with casting linear calcifications are associated with a poorer prognosis.

    e) **False**   Two views are taken for baseline assessment, but single views are usually taken at follow up. Emerging data indicate that two views should be taken in all instances, as this improves lesion detection by up to 40%.

2   a) **True**   A spiculated lesion with central low density on a mammogram may be due to traumatic fat necrosis or radial scar.

    b) **False**   Medullary carcinoma typically presents as a well-defined mass on mammography. Invasive ductal carcinoma is associated with a spiculated mass.

    c) **False**   A phyllodes tumour typically presents as a mass, usually more than 5 cm in size, with lobulated margins. Spiculation is not a prominent feature.

    d) **True**   Other causes of a spiculated lesion on mammography include postsurgical scar, breast abscess, hyalinised fibroadenoma and sclerosing adenosis.

    e) **False**   Plasma cell mastitis is characterised by multiple long linear calcifications on mammography.

3   a) **False**   Cribriform calcifications are typical of low-grade DCIS. High-grade DCIS is associated with casting and branching calcifications.

    b) **True**   Screening mammography has increased the detection of DCIS.

    c) **False**   Although the mammogram is still the most sensitive imaging test in the detection of microcalcifications, DCIS may be recognised on both ultrasonography and MRI. On ultrasonography, casting calcifications of high-grade DCIS result in detectable acoustic shadowing. On MRI, DCIS appears as early linear ductal enhancement following intravenous gadolinium.

    d) **True**   C-erb B-2 oncogene expression is seen in more than 70% of patients with high-grade DCIS. It has also been reported that c-erb B-2 oncogene expression is associated with aggressive histological features and a higher likelihood of rod-shaped and branching calcifications on mammography.

    e) **False**   Lobular carcinoma *in situ* is frequently mammographically occult. The diagnosis is frequently made incidentally on microscopy following surgical resection.

4 a) **False** Medullary carcinoma usually presents as a well-defined mass on the mammogram, which may show a lobulated margin or halo sign. Calcification is not a feature.

b) **True** There is a high incidence of tubular carcinoma in patients with radial scar.

c) **False** Colloid carcinoma, which occurs in an older age group (those over 60 years), is associated with a favourable prognosis because the tumour is slow growing.

d) **False** The most common tumour in the male is still invasive ductal carcinoma. This tends to occur in the subareolar region of the breast.

e) **True** Tumours greater than 1 cm are more likely to metastasise to the axillary lymph nodes.

5 a) **True** Radial scar is a benign proliferative condition, but is associated with an underlying carcinoma (especially tubular carcinoma) in up to 50% of cases. It most frequently presents as an area of parenchymal distortion with a central lucency.

b) **False** The condition is typically bilateral and symmetrical, although it may be unilateral.

c) **True** Lymphoma of the breast is more frequently seen in males and more commonly on the right side.

d) **True** About 85% of metastases to the breast are solitary, usually within the outer upper quadrant. Primary tumours include lymphoma, melanoma, leukaemia and renal cell, lung and ovarian carcinoma. In the male, they may also result from prostatic carcinoma.

e) **True** Galactocoeles appear as well-circumscribed radiolucencies, 1–1.5 cm in size, usually bilateral and multiple. They may be associated with egg-shell calcifications.

6 a) **True** Infiltrated lymph nodes are typically rounded, with a reduced long-to-short axis ratio (normally more than 2).

b) **True** The fatty hilum is frequently obliterated, or there may be eccentric cortical hypertrophy.

c) **True** An increase in resistive index has been reported, which is believed to be the result of compression of the arteries by tumour infiltration.

d) **True** An increase in pulsatility index has also been reported. However, the use of resistive and pulsatility indices has not gained wide acceptance because of conflicting reports in the literature.

e) **True** A peripheral flow pattern is frequently encountered in infiltrated lymph nodes.

7 a) **True** Skin calcifications are recognised by their superficial location and by their lucent centres.

b) **False** On the cranio-caudal view, milk of calcium appears amorphous and ill defined. However, on the medial-lateral oblique view, it is typically sharply defined, semilunar, or crescent-shaped and upwardly concave.

c) **True** Sutural calcification results from calcium deposition on the sutural material. They are typically tubular or linear in appearance and are common in the postirradiated breast.

d) **True** Scattered bilateral calcifications are likely to be benign. However, care should be taken to scrutinise the mammogram for atypical, grouped calcifications.

e) **True** Rim calcification may be seen in the wall of a cyst or surrounding an area of fat necrosis.

8 a) **True** Normal infolding of the implant shell may be seen on MRI as radial folds.
   b) **False** Radial folds are low signal-intensity lines on T2-weighted imaging that arise from the periphery of the implant and are typically thicker than the lines associated with intracapsular rupture, which are made up of two layers of elastomer shell. These folds may be simple or complex.
   c) **False** Intracapsular rupture is more common and is defined as rupture of the elastomer shell with silicone leakage that does not extend beyond the fibrous capsule. Extracapsular rupture results when there is extension of silicone beyond the elastomer shell and fibrous capsule into the breast tissue.
   d) **False** The linguine sign is a reliable indicator of intracapsular rupture, appearing as low-intensity curvilinear lines within the implant.
   e) **True** Gel bleed is the leakage of silicone through microperforations in the implant shell. On MRI, gel bleed may be diagnosed when silicone is seen on both sides of the implant shell (noose or keyhole sign).

9 a) **True** About 65% of fibroadenomas are clinically palpable as discrete but mobile masses.
   b) **False** Although they are multiple in 10%–20% of cases, they are found bilaterally in only about 4%.
   c) **True** Fibroadenomas are common in menstruating women, but tend to regress following the menopause. However, they may continue to be diagnosed in women receiving hormone replacement therapy.
   d) **False** They are well-circumscribed masses, with homogenous internal echoes, but a variable posterior acoustic pattern. Posterior acoustic enhancement is frequently observed.
   e) **True** Nonenhancing internal septations are typically seen within fibroadenomas on gadolinium-enhanced MRI of the breasts.

10 a) **False** They are rare in women under 30 years of age.
   b) **True** They are frequently bilateral and multiple, especially in women with fibrocystic change. Cysts may vary in size and appearance over the course of several months.
   c) **False** Cysts may be aspirated when they are large and symptomatic. However, routine aspiration for cytology is not necessary because intracystic carcinomas are rare.
   d) **False** There is no such evidence.
   e) **True** Cysts containing cellular debris or proteinaceous secretions may show low-level homogenous echoes and may be difficult to distinguish from fibroadenomas. In these cases, aspiration can help to distinguish between the two.

11 a) **True** Linear and punctate calcifications associated with DCIS can be recognised on high-resolution ultrasound as highly reflective foci associated with posterior acoustic shadowing.

b) **True** Invasive ductal carcinoma appears typically as an irregular, poorly marginated hypoechoeic mass, with strong central posterior acoustic shadowing.

c) **True** Posterior acoustic shadowing may arise from the interface of two Cooper's ligaments. The shadowing is typically not associated with a mass and is less apparent or absent if the area is scanned in a plane perpendicular to the initial scan.

d) **True** Extracapsular leakage of silicone results in an area of amorphous reflective echoes.

e) **True** Fibrosis in the surgical scar results in acoustic shadowing.

12 a) **True** A T1 tumour is less than 2 cm in size. T2 denotes a tumour that is greater than 2 cm but less than 5 cm in size. A tumour greater than 5 cm represents T3 disease. A tumour is T4 when there is invasion of the overlying skin or chest wall.

b) **True** Involvement of axillary lymph nodes constitutes N1 disease. Fixed axillary lymph nodes represent N2 disease.

c) **False** Ultrasound tends to underestimate the size of the tumour, as infiltration into adjacent breast tissue may not be visible ultrasonographically.

d) **False** Mammography tends to overestimate the size of the tumour, as it cannot distinguish between tumoural and peritumoural changes.

e) **True** Gadolinium-enhanced MRI is the most sensitive test available for the detection of multicentric and multifocal disease.

13 a) **True** Axillary lymphadenopathy may be seen in association with connective tissue diseases such as systemic lupus erythematosus and scleroderma. Nodal enlargement can also occur in rheumatoid arthritis, granulomatous diseases (e.g. tuberculosis, sarcoidosis), AIDS, infectious mononucleosis, leukaemia and lymphoma.

b) **False** Diabetic fibrous mastopathy is a benign lesion found in patients with type 1 diabetes mellitus that manifests about 20 years after the onset of the disease. It usually presents as a very firm or hard, nontender breast mass in young women.

c) **True** Fibromatosis is a benign, localised, infiltrating mass composed of fibroblasts and collagen. It is typically found in the abdominal wall and, on rare occasions, in the breast. On mammography, it is indistinguishable from an invasive cancer.

d) **True** About 10% of cystosarcoma phyllodes act as malignant tumours.

e) **False** Metastases tend not to cause retraction of the skin or nipple. In addition, metastases are often found in the subcutaneous fat, whereas primary breast cancers develop in the glandular tissue. Metastases usually appear as rounded masses with circumscribed or ill-defined borders. Irregular shape, spiculations and microcalcifications are rare.

14 a) True Sclerosing adenosis occurs as part of a spectrum of proliferative abnormalities referred to as fibrocystic change. It may be focal or diffuse, appearing as a focal cluster of microcalcifications or as diffuse calcifications on mammography, and it may be associated with a spiculated mass.

   b) False It is associated with only a mild (2.5-fold) increase in the risk of infiltrating breast cancer. The condition itself is nonmalignant.

   c) True At mammography, sclerosing adenosis forms part of a differential diagnosis for spiculated lesions that includes both malignant and benign conditions. The diagnosis is often only made following biopsy.

   d) False Although sclerosing adenosis may manifest as a clinically palpable mass (adenosis tumour), it is frequently only detected on mammography.

   e) True Lobular carcinoma *in situ* may be found in areas of sclerosing adenosis.

15 a) False Fat necrosis is most common in obese, usually middle-aged women with fatty, pendulous breasts.

   b) True It usually occurs in the superficial aspect of the breast.

   c) True The most common causes are surgery and radiation treatment, although it may result from trauma.

   d) False The mammographic spectrum of fat necrosis ranges from clearly benign, through indeterminate, to malignant-appearing masses or calcifications. Skin retraction may be a feature.

   e) True Calcifications may be curvilinear, punctate or show central lucencies.

16 a) False Postoperative fluid collections are identified in 50% of patients at 4 weeks and in 25% of patients at 6 months following surgery. Most fluid collections resolve by 12 months. They appear as oval, dense, well-defined masses with minimal spiculation.

   b) True Parenchymal scarring is characterised by the absence of a central mass, a changing appearance on different projections and thick, curvilinear spicules. A soft-tissue density interspersed with radiolucent areas representing entrapped fat is typical.

   c) False Benign calcifications, including needle-like calcifications, thick calcified plaques and thin arcs of calcium around radiolucent oil cysts, may occur 2–44 months after breast conservation therapy. However, the appearance of new microcalcification would raise suspicion of local recurrence.

   d) True This is due to radiation-induced oedema.

   e) False Maximal skin thickening is usually identified in the first 6 months after completion of radiation therapy. This gradually resolves over 2–3 years.

17 a) **True** This is one of the most important roles of ultrasonography.
   b) **True** A palpable abnormality can be scrutinised using ultrasound. However, a palpable abnormality may be invisible on both ultrasonography and mammography. Note that ultrasonography has a very high false-negative rate (up to 40%) in the detection of cancer.
   c) **True** Mastitis not responding to appropriate antibiotics may be evaluated using ultrasonography to detect a possible underlying abscess.
   d) **False** Ultrasonography in young women should also be guided by the presence of any palpable abnormality, although it is not uncommon for surgeons and clinicians to request the test to assuage a patient's anxiety.
   e) **False** Ultrasonography is not routinely used in the evaluation of an asymptomatic dense breast.

18 a) **False** Biopsy in the breast is usually performed with 14G cutting needles.
   b) **True** Typically, 10 or more cores of tissues are obtained from an area of suspected microcalcifications.
   c) **False** The pair of mammographic images is typically 15° off-centre on either side. This allows the machine to generate the co-ordinates for the biopsy.
   d) **True** Specimen radiography is essential to verify that the core specimens contain microcalcifications. The presence of microcalcifications within the specimen increases the likelihood of a definitive diagnosis.
   e) **True** Mammotomy uses a cutter connected to a suction device, which allows quick and easy sampling. Tissue samples are harvested without removing the device from the breast.

19 a) **True** This is typically well defined with a fatty hilum.
   b) **True** This solitary intraductal papilloma usually occurs in the subareolar region. They are usually small and mammographically occult, but may grow to present as a circumscribed lesion.
   c) **True** A galactocoele may appear as a well-defined, fat-containing lesion.
   d) **True** Lipomas are fat containing and well defined.
   e) **True** Haematomas are typically ill defined initially, but become better defined as they mature and organise. Most of these resolve completely, but some may result in focal calcifications.

20 a) **False** The halo sign may be seen in invasive cancers.
   b) **False** MRI is often performed during this window (the second week of the menstrual cycle). The normal breast tissue can enhance significantly with intravenous gadolinium about a week before menstruation and may obscure an underlying lesion.
   c) **False** The normal nipple and subareolar tissue enhance avidly with intravenous gadolinium. MRI is therefore insensitive in the detection of Paget's disease of the nipple.
   d) **True** Cancers may show early peripheral enhancement with more delayed central enhancement.
   e) **True** This is the typical appearance of cancers on dynamic gadolinium-enhanced MRI. However, some benign lesions (e.g. fibroadenoma) may uncommonly demonstrate this appearance.

178

Chapter 10

Interventional radiology

1   **Regarding local anaesthesia, which of the following are true?**
    a) Toxic effects from subcutaneous lignocaine usually occur within 10 minutes
        of administration
    b) Circumoral tingling is an early sign of toxicity
    c) 10 ml of 1% lignocaine contains 50 mg of lignocaine
    d) The maximum nontoxic dose of lignocaine for a 70 kg man is 200 mg
    e) Lignocaine is effectively absorbed through mucous membranes

?   **Regarding sedation, which of the following are true?**
    a) Midazolam causes a fall in blood pressure
    b) Flumazenil is a benzodiazepine
    c) The elimination half-life of flumazenil is longer than that of midazolam
    d) Midazolam shows minimal protein binding
    e) The amnesia produced by diazepam is more predictable than by midazolam

3   **Indications for percutaneous embolisation include which of the following?**
    a) Postpartum haemorrhage
    b) Juvenile nasopharyngeal angiofibroma
    c) Acoustic neuroma
    d) Haemoptysis
    e) Carotid–cavernous sinus fistulae

4   **Regarding transjugular intrahepatic porto-systemic shunts (TIPS), which
    of the following are true?**
    a) The aim is to produce a porto-systemic shunt gradient of approximately 5 mm Hg
    b) Embolisation of varices can be performed as part of the procedure
    c) Right-sided heart failure is a relative contraindication
    d) About 20% of stents have occluded at 1 year
    e) Ultrasound is accurate in the assessment of shunt patency

5   **Regarding peripheral thrombolysis, which of the following are true?**
    a) Tissue plasminogen activator (tPA) converts plasminogen to plasmin,
        which promotes clot lysis
    b) tPA is contraindicated in patients with a recent history of transient ischaemic
        attacks (within 6 months)
    c) Following tPA, angioplasty should be deferred for 24 hours
    d) tPA is typically combined with systemic intravenous heparin
    e) The patient's blood pressure, pulse rate and puncture site should be checked
        hourly following initiation of thrombolysis

6   **Regarding adrenal vein sampling in the assessment of hyperaldosteronism,
    which of the following are true?**
    a) Samples from both adrenal veins are taken simultaneously
    b) The left adrenal vein is harder to cannulate than the right
    c) Samples are taken before and 1 hour after administration of synthetic
        adrenocorticotrophic hormone (ACTH)
    d) Adrenal vein sampling is the most reliable method for distinguishing a unilateral
        aldosterone-secreting adenoma from bilateral hyperplasia
    e) Adrenal venography is routinely performed during adrenal vein sampling

7   **Which of the following are true regarding the bronchial arteries?**
   a)   The bronchial arteries most commonly arise from the descending aorta at the T5/T6 level
   b)   The bronchial arteries also supply blood to the oesophagus
   c)   The most common cause of massive haemoptysis in the developed world
        is bronchogenic carcinoma
   d)   When searching for a cause of massive haemoptysis, the subclavian arteries
        should be examined
   e)   Rasmussen's aneurysm arises from the bronchial arteries

8   **Regarding percutaneous transhepatic cholangiography (PTC) and biliary drainage,
    which of the following are true?**
   a)   A contraindication to percutaneous biliary drainage is obstruction complicated
        by cholangitis and septicaemia
   b)   PTC is to be avoided in the presence of a large amount of ascites
   c)   Punctured lymphatic vessels are recognised by their smooth, tapered appearance
        on injecting a contrast agent
   d)   Bacteraemia occurs more commonly during diagnostic PTC than during
        percutaneous biliary drainage
   e)   A bilious pleural effusion may occur following successful biliary drainage

9   **Regarding uterine artery embolisation (UAE), which of the following are true?**
   a)   Coils are the embolisation agent of choice
   b)   The uterine arteries anastomose with the ovarian arteries
   c)   Pain typically begins 6–8 hours after the procedure
   d)   The quoted risk of infection needing a hysterectomy following UAE is 0.1%
   e)   Sarcomatous change within a fibroid uterus is readily diagnosed on magnetic
        resonance imaging (MRI)

10 **Which of the following statements are true?**
   a)   Nitinol is an alloy composed of steel and titanium
   b)   Nitinol is more radio-opaque than stainless steel
   c)   Stent grafts are usually covered in polytetrafluoroethylene (PTFE)
   d)   Neointimal hyperplasia refers to excess endothelial cells in the vessel intima
   e)   Covered stents produce greater neointimal hyperplasia than bare metal stents

11 **Regarding superior vena cava obstruction (SVCO), which of the following are true?**
   a)   SVCO is often successfully treated with balloon angioplasty
   b)   Radiotherapy is the first-line treatment in malignant SVCO
   c)   In stenting SVCO, the femoral approach is preferred
   d)   Thrombolysis is rarely useful
   e)   Migration of superior vena cava stents into the right side of the heart
        is a common complication

12 **Regarding percutaneous gastrostomy, which of the following are true?**
   a)   Prophylactic antibiotics are routinely used
   b)   Ascites is a relative contraindication
   c)   The gastric fundus is the preferred site of puncture
   d)   Feeding should only be started via the gastrostomy tube after 1 week
   e)   Gastropexy with 'T-fasteners' prior to insertion of the gastrostomy tube reduces
        the complication rate

13 **Regarding Doppler ultrasound of peripheral arteries, which of the following are true?**
   a) Triphasic blood flow in a normal artery implies a high-resistance distal vascular bed
   b) Spectral broadening occurs in a normal vessel supplying a low-resistance vascular bed
   c) The resistive index is calculated from the maximum systolic velocity minus the maximum end diastolic velocity divided by the maximum systolic velocity
   d) In the majority of patients, the internal carotid artery (ICA) is postero-medial to the external carotid artery (ECA)
   e) Power Doppler is independent of the angle of the incident ultrasound waves on the vessel

14 **Regarding fibromuscular dysplasia (FMD), which of the following are true?**
   a) It characteristically affects the mid and distal main renal artery
   b) It most commonly affects the vessel intima
   c) Renal FMD is usually bilateral
   d) Transluminal angioplasty has a high long-term success rate in renal FMD
   e) FMD also affects the mesenteric vessels

15 **Regarding endoscopic ultrasound (EUS), which of the following are true?**
   a) Five separate layers are identified on EUS of the oesophagus
   b) EUS can distinguish different echogenicities of the ventral and dorsal pancreas
   c) Involvement of the muscularis propia implies tumour spread through the oesophageal wall
   d) Fine needle aspiration of lesions lying outside the bowel lumen can be performed during EUS
   e) The liver is not visualised on EUS

16 **Regarding the risks of lung biopsy, which of the following are true?**
   a) Pneumothoraces occur in 15%–25% of patients with chronic obstructive pulmonary disease (COPD) following percutaneous lung biopsy
   b) Following percutaneous lung biopsy, the patient should be observed for 1 hour prior to discharge
   c) Haemoptysis should be managed by placing the patient in a lateral decubitus position with the biopsied lung dependent
   d) Pleural masses are best biopsied under ultrasound control
   e) When performing an anterior mediastinal biopsy, the internal mammary arteries can be avoided by using a puncture site greater than 1 cm from the sternal edge

17 **In hepatic angiography, which of the following produce hypervascular liver lesions?**
   a) Breast cancer metastases
   b) Islet cell pancreatic metastases
   c) Renal cell metastases
   d) Colonic metastases
   e) Ovarian cystadenocarcinoma metastases

18 **Regarding varicocoele embolisation, which of the following are true?**
   a) The procedure can be performed from either a femoral vein or internal jugular vein approach
   b) Complications of the procedure include hydrocele formation
   c) Testicular infarction is a recognised complication
   d) Gelfoam is a suitable embolisation agent
   e) The relationship between infertility and varicoceles is well defined

19 **Regarding pulmonary arteriovenous malformations (PAVMs), which of the following are true?**
   a) PAVMs cause a left-to-right shunt
   b) The majority of patients have hereditary haemorrhagic telangiectasia
   c) The majority of PAVMs occur in the lower lobes
   d) Polyvinyl alcohol particles are the embolising agent of choice
   e) Multiple PAVMs are more common than solitary lesions

20 **Regarding percutaneous nephrostomy, which of the following are true?**
   a) A direct puncture of the renal pelvis is recommended
   b) Complete renal obstruction requires urgent decompression
   c) Colonic injury does not occur with a postero-lateral approach
   d) Pseudoaneurysms within the kidney can be treated with angiographic embolisation
   e) Percutaneous removal in combination with extracorporeal lithotripsy is the first-line treatment for calyceal stones

21 **Regarding intra-arterial heparin bolus, which of the following are true?**
   a) It is indicated for renal artery stent placement
   b) It is indicated for iliac artery angioplasty
   c) It is indicated for posterior tibial artery angioplasty
   d) It is indicated for embolisation of a renal pseudoaneurysm
   e) A repeat intra-arterial lesion bolus is indicated if the procedure exceeds 2 hours

22 **Regarding cholecystostomy, which of the following are true?**
   a) A direct puncture of the gallbladder is the preferred method
   b) An empyema is a contraindication
   c) It is of no benefit in acalculous cholecystitis
   d) Gallstone extraction can be performed via the cholecystostomy once the tract has been left to mature for 1–2 weeks
   e) Antibiotic cover should be given in all cases

23 **Regarding interventional procedures of the liver, which of the following are true?**
   a) Severe coagulopathy is a contraindication to transjugular liver biopsy
   b) Subdiaphragmatic lesions are best biopsied under computed tomography (CT) guidance
   c) Aspiration or drainage of suspected hydatid cysts is contraindicated
   d) Shoulder pain is common following liver biopsy
   e) A transhepatic route can be used to biopsy the right adrenal gland

24 **Regarding the subclavian steal syndrome, which of the following are true?**
   a) It results from stenosis of the proximal subclavian artery
   b) It is more common on the left side
   c) The diagnosis can be made on Doppler ultrasound
   d) Percutaneous angioplasty offers good long-term results
   e) Atherosclerosis is the most common cause of subclavian steal

25 **Regarding Behçet's disease, which of the following are true?**
   a) It typically has a relapsing course
   b) Erythema multiforme is a feature
   c) It is a cause of pulmonary artery aneurysm
   d) It is a cause of SVCO
   e) It is a cause of destructive arthritis

26 **Regarding angiodysplasia, which of the following are true?**
   a) It is most commonly seen in the caecum and ascending colon
   b) It is associated with mitral valve disease
   c) Angiography should not be performed in haemodynamically unstable patients
   d) Gastrointestinal bleeding can be detected by angiography only if the rate of bleeding is ≥ 0.1 ml/min
   e) It typically presents with severe gastrointestinal bleeding

27 **Regarding hysterosalpingography, which of the following are true?**
   a) Opacification of the ovarian and iliac veins is inconsequential
   b) A pregnancy test should be performed before every examination
   c) The Fallopian tube is narrowest in its intramural segment
   d) Uterus didelphys implies complete separation of the uterine body down to the internal os
   e) Salpingitis isthmica nodosa causes irregularity of the uterine cavity

28 **Regarding aortic stent grafting, which of the following are true?**
   a) Endoleaks due to retrograde filling of the aneurysm sac from side-branches require urgent treatment
   b) Stent migration is a common problem
   c) If the aneurysm extends down into the pelvis to involve an internal iliac artery, then stent grafting is not feasible
   d) Endoleaks can only be detected by repeat angiography
   e) Stent grafts can be used for aortic arch aneurysms

29 **Regarding popliteal artery entrapment syndrome, which of the following are true?**
   a) It typically occurs in young men
   b) The syndrome presents with progressive intermittent claudication
   c) The condition is secondary to compression of the popliteal artery by the medial head of the gastrocnemius
   d) Angiography is frequently unhelpful
   e) The condition is often bilateral

30 **Regarding traumatic rupture of the aorta, which of the following are true?**
   a) The most common site is just proximal to the origin of the left subclavian artery
   b) Superior displacement of the left main-stem bronchus is typically seen
   c) About 20% of patients with a traumatic rupture will die before reaching hospital
   d) Dysphagia is a presenting symptom
   e) A normal CT scan excludes the diagnosis of an aortic rupture

31 In acute Budd–Chiari syndrome, which of the following are true?
a) Hepatofugal flow within the main portal vein is typical
b) A hepatic venogram is not possible
c) An enlarged enhancing caudate lobe is seen on contrast-enhanced CT
d) Stenting of the inferior vena cava (IVC) is a recognised treatment
e) There is an association with paroxysmal nocturnal haemoglobinuria

32 Regarding stenting of the iliac arteries for atherosclerotic disease, which of the following are true?
a) A postangioplasty residual systolic pressure gradient of greater than 15 mm Hg requires stenting
b) The 5-year patency rate of iliac artery stenting is 70%–75%
c) Stenting is always required if intimal dissection occurs following angioplasty
d) Delayed stent occlusion is usually due to thrombosis at the mouth of the stent
e) Stenting of both common iliac arteries should be performed for a proximal unilateral common iliac stenosis

33 Glucagon is contraindicated in the presence of which of the following?
a) Insulinoma
b) Cardiac arrhythmia
c) Phaeochromocytoma
d) Diabetes mellitus
e) Glucagonoma

34 Regarding mesenteric angiography, which of the following are true?
a) The superior mesenteric artery should be evaluated before the inferior mesenteric artery (IMA)
b) Vasopressin can be used to control colonic bleeding
c) Upper gastrointestinal haemorrhage should be initially treated using endoscopic techniques
d) The IMA arises at the level of the L4 vertebral body
e) Diverticular haemorrhage is the most common cause of colonic bleeding

35 Regarding oesophageal stents, which of the following are true?
a) Following oesophageal stenting, central chest pain occurs in 50% of cases
b) Stent migration is more common with covered oesophageal stents
c) Sedation is usually required for oesophageal stent placement
d) Balloon rupture during balloon dilatation of an oesophageal stricture is associated with a high rate of oesophageal tears
e) Stenting is preferred to balloon dilatation for the treatment of achalasia

36 Regarding colonic stents, which of the following are true?
a) Colonic stents provide good long-term palliation for colonic tumours
b) Covered stents are typically used when treating colonic tumours
c) Stents can be deployed throughout the colon
d) Colonic stents should not be used to treat benign disease
e) Antibiotic cover is routinely required before colonic stenting

37 Regarding transrectal ultrasound (TRUS) of the prostate, which of the following are true?
  a) TRUS is the most accurate method of detecting prostatic carcinoma
  b) With TRUS, the peripheral zone is echogenic compared to the central zone
  c) Prostatic carcinoma usually appears hyperechoic on TRUS
  d) Antibiotic cover is always required for a TRUS-guided prostatic biopsy
  e) Two or three cores of tissue should be taken from the peripheral zone of the gland

38 Which of the following statements are true?
  a) Occlusion of a large arteriovenous fistula results in immediate tachycardia
  b) Dissecting aneurysms confined to the descending thoracic aorta require urgent surgical intervention
  c) Dissecting aneurysms of the ascending aorta occur in Marfan's syndrome
  d) A double superior vena cava is seen more frequently than an isolated left-sided SVC
  e) Fibrosing mediastinitis is caused by histiocytosis

39 Which of the following statements are true?
  a) Renal angiomyolipomas appear vascular at arteriography
  b) Transverse myelitis is a complication of bronchial arteriography
  c) Fibrosing mediastinitis often results in SVCO
  d) A bleeding Meckel's diverticulum is best diagnosed using mesenteric angiography
  e) Small-bowel leiomyomas may be diagnosed on arteriography

40 Which of the following are true regarding renal artery stenosis (RAS)?
  a) RAS is associated with type 1 neurofibromatosis (NF-1)
  b) RAS following renal transplantation typically involves a long segment of the artery
  c) Renal artery stent placement is usually required for ostial stenoses
  d) Renovascular disease accounts for approximately 15% of all cases of hypertension
  e) Extravasation of contrast from the renal artery following angioplasty requires urgent surgery

Answers

1 a) **False** Maximum arterial plasma concentrations of lignocaine develop between 10 and 25 minutes following administration.
   b) **True** This can progress to confusion, hypotension, respiratory depression and convulsions.
   c) **False** 1% lignocaine contains 10 mg/ml of the drug.
   d) **True** This corresponds to 20 ml of 1% lignocaine.
   e) **True** Concentrations of up to 4% provide good surface anaesthesia.

2 a) **True** This is due to a reduction in systemic vascular resistance.
   b) **True** Flumazenil is a specific benzodiazepine antagonist. Its affinity for receptors is good, resulting in displacement of sedative benzodiazepines and reversal of sedation.
   c) **False** The elimination half-life is shorter (50–60 minutes) than that of midazolam. Repeat doses may be required to maintain the reversal of sedative benzodiazepines.
   d) **False** Midazolam is 90% protein bound. Increased effects may be seen in patients with low plasma albumin levels.
   e) **False** The amnesia produced by midazolam is more predictable than that produced by diazepam.

3 a) **True** The percutaneous embolisation procedure will often avoid the need for a hysterectomy following postpartum haemorrhage.
   b) **True** This highly vascular tumour is often embolised preoperatively to reduce blood loss during surgery. Highly selective embolisation is required.
   c) **False** This tumour may be highly vascular, but embolisation is not usually feasible.
   d) **True** The bronchial arteries are the usual source of haemoptysis.
   e) **True** This is the treatment of choice for spontaneous carotid–cavernous sinus fistulae, using either detachable balloons or coils. Posttraumatic fistulae can be treated conservatively.

4 a) **False** A TIPS procedure is indicated in patients with variceal bleeding despite sclerotherapy or endoscopic banding, patients with varices inaccessible to endoscopy and in those at high risk of bleeding whilst awaiting liver transplantation. Less commonly, TIPS is used in the treatment of rapid onset ascites or the treatment of Budd–Chiari syndrome. The aim is to produce a porto-systemic shunt gradient of 10–15 mm Hg, which is usually sufficient to reduce variceal bleeding and avoid the risk of encephalopathy.
   b) **True** Actively bleeding varices can be embolised with coils via the porto-systemic shunt.
   c) **True** This is due to right heart pressure being transmitted through the shunt into the portal system.
   d) **False** Stent occlusion, due to intimal hyperplasia, reaches 50% at 1 year. Early complications include extracapsular portal vein damage, haemobilia, sepsis and encephalopathy.
   e) **True** Doppler ultrasound is the imaging modality of choice in assessing shunt patency.

5 a) **True** tPA converts plasminogen to plasmin, which lyses fibrin to dissolve thrombus.

   b) **False** tPA is contraindicated if there is a history of a cerebrovascular accident within 6 months, but only contraindicated if the procedure is within 2 months of a transient ischaemic attack.

   c) **False** Underlying stenoses are often uncovered by tPA, resulting in the need for percutaneous angioplasty. This can be performed immediately following tPA.

   d) **True** Evidence *in vitro* suggests that the combination of heparin and tPA is more effective than tPA alone.

   e) **False** These parameters should be checked at 15-minute intervals for the first hour and then hourly until the thrombosis is stopped. The patient should ideally be nursed on a high-dependency unit.

6 a) **True** Because the secretion of aldosterone by an adenoma is pulsatile, simultaneous sampling from both sides is essential. This may be performed via bilateral femoral vein punctures.

   b) **False** The right adrenal vein drains directly into the IVC and is shorter than the left, which drains into the left renal vein. This makes the right side more difficult to cannulate.

   c) **False** Samples are taken 15 minutes after the ACTH infusion has started. In patients with an aldosterone-secreting adrenal adenoma, there will be an abrupt increase in cortisol and aldosterone levels from the side of the adenoma. On the normal side, only the cortisol levels will rise.

   d) **True** CT scanning can detect adrenal nodules greater than 7 mm in diameter. Adrenal vein sampling has almost 100% accuracy in detecting any size of adenoma.

   e) **False** CT scanning is superior to venography at demonstrating adrenal nodules. In addition, venography carries the risk of adrenal infarction and is therefore not performed.

7 a) **True** The most common configuration is with a single artery arising on the right and two arteries arising on the left. Many variations of this have been described.

   b) **True** The bronchial arteries also supply the diaphragmatic and mediastinal visceral pleura, the vasa vasora of the aorta, pulmonary arteries and, occasionally, the myocardium and spinal cord.

   c) **False** Chronic suppuration, usually due to bronchiectasis, is the most common cause of massive haemoptysis in the developed world. Aspergillomas within chronic tuberculosis (TB) cavities are also more common than bronchogenic carcinoma as a cause of massive haemoptysis.

   d) **True** Subclavian artery branches via transpleural vessels may contribute blood supply to the chronically inflamed lung. Other nonbronchial arteries that may supply systemic blood to the lung include the intercostal arteries, the axillary arteries and the inferior phrenic arteries.

   e) **False** This rare aneurysm arises from the pulmonary arterial tree secondary to erosion from adjacent lung disease (commonly TB).

8 a) **False** In combination with antibiotics, PTC is the treatment of choice.

b) **True** If possible, the ascites should be drained first to avoid the increased risk of intraperitoneal haemorrhage or bile peritonitis.

c) **False** Intrahepatic lymphatic vessels have a characteristic beaded appearance. Injection into the portal and hepatic veins is recognised by the rapid flow of contrast in a direction away from the liver hilum. Contrast injected into the biliary tree flows much more slowly away from the needle tip.

d) **True** Bacteraemia, possibly complicated by endotoxic shock, is a result of increasing the pressure in the biliary tree during injection of contrast medium.

e) **True** A biliary catheter can traverse the parietal pleura, resulting in a bile effusion.

9 a) **False** Polyvinyl alcohol particles are typically used. Gelatin sponge particles have also been shown to be effective. Coils as the sole embolisation agent do not effectively embolise the small uterine vessels and are therefore not recommended.

b) **True** This can result in particles embolising the ovaries, with the associated risk of ovarian failure and early menopause. This is reported to occur in 1% of cases, although it appears more likely to occur in the older patient.

c) **False** Pain usually begins as soon as the second uterine artery has been embolised.

d) **False** The reported rate of hysterectomy following UAE is 1%–2%. This is slightly higher in patients with very large fibroids.

e) **False** The diagnosis of sarcomatous change is difficult with any imaging modality. Rapid growth within a fibroid should raise suspicions, although this can be seen in benign fibroids. Histology should be obtained if there are any concerns. Fortunately, sarcomatous change is extremely rare.

10 a) **False** Nitinol is an alloy composed chiefly of nickel and titanium. Its properties include a thermal memory and superelasticity, making it ideal for stent manufacture.

b) **False** The reverse is true.

c) **True** Dacron or polyurethane are also used.

d) **False** Neointimal hyperplasia refers to the proliferation and migration of vascular smooth muscle cells and extracellular matrix from the media into the intima following trauma to the vessel wall.

e) **True** The exact reasons for this are unclear. It may be due to the larger foreign area of a stent graft causing a larger thrombogenic response. Dacron in particular produces a local inflammatory response in the vessel wall, with release of cytokines and possible promotion of neointimal hyperplasia.

11 a) **False** Recurrence rates are high as the underlying aetiology is often outside the SVC. However, angioplasty combined with stenting is a treatment option.

b) **True** There is often a rapid response to malignant SVCO following radiotherapy, especially in the case of lymphoma. Malignant causes account for greater than 80% of cases. Benign causes include aortic aneurysms, thyroid goitres and TB mediastinitis.

c) **True** The femoral vein usually provides the best approach.

d) **False** Thrombolysis helps to identify the underlying stenosis within the vessel, often prior to insertion of a stent.

e) **False** Migration of stents into the right side of the heart, occasionally as far as the pulmonary artery, is a rare but recognised complication.

12 a) **False** Antibiotics are not indicated.

    b) **True** Ascites may prevent maturation of the catheter tract, resulting in leak of stomach contents into the peritoneum or a percutaneous ascitic leak.

    c) **False** The preferred puncture site lies inferior to the left lobe of the liver, midway between the greater and lesser curves and at the junction of the upper two thirds and lower one third of the stomach.

    d) **False** Providing the patient shows no signs of peritonitis, the gastrostomy tube can be used after 24 hours.

    e) **False** 'T-fasteners' reduce the risk of catheter displacement into the peritoneum. They do, however, increase the risk of gastric wall pressure necrosis. Overall, the complication rate is reported to be little altered whether or not 'T-fasteners' are used. Most centres routinely use 'T-fasteners'.

13 a) **True** This is due to a combination of an elastic vessel wall and a high-resistance distal vascular bed, such as the superficial femoral artery with the leg at rest.

    b) **False** Spectral broadening implies blood flow of different velocities within an artery. This is commonly seen around an arterial stenosis due to turbulent flow.

    c) **True** The resistive index is useful in detecting changes in downstream vascular resistance.

    d) **False** The ICA is positioned postero-lateral to the ECA.

    e) **True** This is in contrast to colour Doppler ultrasound, which is angle dependent. Thus, power Doppler gives no information about direction or velocity of flow.

14 a) **True** The proximal third of the renal artery is typically affected by atherosclerosis, but rarely by FMD.

    b) **False** The media is affected in 60%–85% of cases. Medial fibroplasia is characterised by a 'string of beads' appearance of alternating stenoses and aneurysms within the mid and distal main renal artery.

    c) **True** It is bilateral in two thirds of cases.

    d) **True** Low restenosis rates have been reported. Atherosclerotic disease often requires stenting due to high restenosis rates.

    e) **True** FMD affects other vessels in 1%–2% of cases. These include the celiac, hepatic, splenic, mesenteric, iliac and internal carotid vessels.

15 a) **True** Five layers can be identified. The first layer (echogenic) corresponds to the mucosal surface, the second (echopoor) to the muscularis mucosa, the third (echogenic) to the submucosa, the fourth (echopoor) to the muscularis propria and the fifth (echogenic) to the serosa.

    b) **True** The dorsal pancreas may appear hypoechoic compared to the ventral pancreas.

    c) **True** This is easily identified on EUS, resulting in accurate local staging.

    d) **True** Fine needle aspiration can be performed safely on lesions outside the bowel wall. This includes lymph nodes and solid organs, such as the liver and pancreas.

    e) **False** A large proportion of the liver is clearly identified on EUS.

16 a) **False** Pneumothoraces occur in 50% of patients with COPD. In patients with no underlying diffuse lung disease, pneumothoraces occur in 15%–25% of cases.

b) **False** Most practitioners agree that patients should be observed for at least 4 hours before being discharged. This allows day-case procedures to be performed. An erect chest X-ray is usually performed before discharge.

c) **True** This will prevent blood being aspirated into the contralateral lung.

d) **True** Ultrasound is faster and cheaper than CT and may reduce the risk of a pneumothorax by showing, and hence allowing avoidance of, the interface between the pleura and the lung during biopsy. This clearly does not apply to pleural masses within the fissures.

e) **False** The internal mammary arteries descend behind the costal cartilages, approximately 1.25 cm lateral to the sternal edge.

17 All true Other tumours with hypervascular liver metastases include carcinoid, melanoma, choriocarcinoma, sarcoma and phaeochromocytoma.

18 a) **True** The internal jugular vein approach is often preferred as it allows a more favourable angle of approach to the testicular vein.

b) **False** Complications are rare and include migration of embolic material to the lung and thrombophlebitis of the pampiniform plexus.

c) **False** See b).

d) **False** Coils, detachable balloons or sclerosing agents are the recognised occluding agents. Particulate embolic material is not recommended.

e) **False** There is still debate about the role of varicocele embolisation in the treatment of infertility.

19 a) **False** PAVMs are congenital communications between the pulmonary artery and pulmonary vein causing a right-to-left shunt.

b) **True** This is Osler–Weber–Rendu syndrome. Approximately 50%–80% of patients have this condition, although only 15% of patients with Osler–Weber–Rendu syndrome have PAVMs.

c) **True** Most (60%–70%) occur in the lower lobes.

d) **False** Particles may pass into the systemic circulation. Coils or detachable balloons are the agents of choice.

e) **False** Single lesions are seen in two thirds of patients.

20 a) **False** A transparenchymal renal tract is preferred, as it reduces the risk of tearing the renal pelvis and of damaging a major renal vessel.

b) **False** Urgent intervention is only required if an obstructed kidney is complicated by the presence of infection.

c) **False** A retrorenal colon is a recognised normal variant and therefore can be punctured via a postero-lateral approach. It may be difficult to identify prospectively. It is thought to be more common in thinner patients.

d) **True** Renal haemorrhage following percutaneous nephrostomy is the most common complication. Arteriovenous fistulae and pseudoaneurysms have been reported in 0.5%–1% of cases and often require embolisation as treatment.

e) **False** Extracorporeal lithotripsy alone is the first-line treatment for calyceal stones in the majority of patients.

21 a) **True** Antispasmodics may also be required.
   b) **False** The high flow in the iliac vessels makes heparin unnecessary.
   c) **True** Heparin is required for any angioplasty within the lower limb.
   d) **False**
   e) **False** If the procedure exceeds a maximum of 1 hour, a repeat bolus is required as heparin has a short half-life.

22 a) **False** A transhepatic puncture is preferred in the hope of reducing the chance of an intraperitoneal bile leak.
   b) **False** An empyema is one of the main indications for the procedure, especially in patients unfit for a general anaesthetic.
   c) **False** Cholecystostomy has been reported as beneficial in acalculous cholecystitis, especially in critically ill patients in an intensive care unit.
   d) **False** The tract should be allowed to mature for at least 4–6 weeks.
   e) **True** This is true for all percutaneous transhepatic biliary procedures because of the high risk of cholangitis.

23 a) **False** Severe coagulopathy is an indication for the transjugular route.
   b) **False** Ultrasound guidance is preferred, as it is easier to compensate for respiratory motion with this method.
   c) **False** It is now felt that there is only a minimal risk of anaphylaxis or dissemination of cysts following percutaneous intervention.
   d) **True** This is due to referred pain from irritation of the diaphragm.
   e) **True** The liver often provides a good ultrasound 'window' to view the adrenal gland.

24 a) **True** The subclavian artery stenosis causes blood flow to be reversed in the ipsilateral vertebral artery, in order to provide blood flow to the arm. This is particularly seen when the arm is exercised and results in signs of vertebro-basilar insufficiency.
   b) **True** It is three times more common on the left side than the right side.
   c) **True** Doppler ultrasound may show reversal of flow in the vertebral artery on exercising the arm. The subclavian artery stenosis may be difficult to demonstrate.
   d) **True** Stenting is rarely required.
   e) **True** Other causes include preductal infantile coarctation, hypoplasia of the left aortic arch, a dissecting aneurysm, trauma and radiation fibrosis.

25 a) **True** It is a systemic vasculitis of unknown cause, characterised by oral ulceration, genital ulceration and iritis.
   b) **False** Erythema nodosum is a feature.
   c) **True** These may erode into the bronchial tree, causing massive haemoptysis.
   d) **True** This is due to SVC thrombosis. Thromboembolism is also seen in this disease.
   e) **False** It causes a mild, nondestructive arthritis.

26 a) **True**   Only 25% of cases involve the descending and sigmoid colon.

     b) **False**   However, it is associated with aortic stenosis in 20% of cases.

     c) **False**   Urgent angiography is indicated in haemodynamically unstable patients, as the site of bleeding is more likely to be identified. Stable patients should first undergo nuclear medicine imaging.

     d) **False**   Sulphur colloid scanning will detect gastrointestinal bleeding at a rate of 0.05–0.1 ml/min. Angiography is much less sensitive, requiring a bleeding rate of at least 0.5 ml/min.

     e) **False**   Angiodysplasia usually presents with anaemia due to chronic blood loss.

27 a) **True**   Venous intravasation itself is of little importance, although it does imply increased pressure of contrast within the uterine cavity. This may be due to tubal disease, menstruation, intrauterine synechia, uterine anomalies or excessive injection pressure.

     b) **False**   To avoid radiation of an early pregnancy the examination should be performed before ovulation. If there is any doubt, a pregnancy test should be performed.

     c) **False**   The Fallopian tube is divided into four parts: intramural, isthmus, ampulla and fimbria. The isthmus is the narrowest segment.

     d) **False**   Didelphys implies complete duplication of the uterus, cervical os and vagina. When separation occurs down to the external os, it is termed 'uterus bicornuate bicollis'.

     e) **False**   As the name suggests, salpingitis isthmica nodosa causes irregularity of the isthmic portion of the Fallopian tube. This is associated with small diverticula and may progress to obstruction. It is clinically important because of the common association with pelvic inflammatory disease, infertility and ectopic pregnancy.

28 a) **False**   Endoleaks occur when blood fills the space between the stent graft and the original aneurysm sac, causing continued expansion of the aneurysm. There are two broad categories of endoleak – those related to the endograft itself, including the anastomoses or fixation sites (types 1 and 3), and those due to retrograde flow into the aneurysm sac from patent aortic side branches (type 2). Types 1 and 3 should be treated urgently, whereas type 2 endoleaks can be managed with continued surveillance.

     b) **False**   The early stents migrated frequently. With more recent designs, however, stent migration is an uncommon problem.

     c) **False**   In this situation, the internal iliac artery is embolised before stent-graft placement to prevent retrograde flow into the aneurysm sac.

     d) **False**   Arterial phase helical CT has been shown to be an effective method of radiological surveillance to detect leaks.

     e) **True**   Branching aortic stent grafts have been deployed successfully in the aortic arch.

29 a) True It is nine times more common in men than women and two thirds of patients are under 35 years of age.

b) **True** Pain typically occurs during prolonged standing or following vigorous exercise.

c) **True** The popliteal artery is located medially and deep to the medial head of the gastrocnemius.

d) **False** In the resting position, the popliteal artery may appear normal or show slight medial deviation. The diagnosis is made after active plantar flexion of the foot against resistance. Angiography shows an abrupt cut-off of the popliteal artery at the level of the medial head of the gastrocnemius. This may be complicated by a poststenotic aneurysm.

e) **True** Up to two thirds of patients have this syndrome in both legs.

30 a) False About 90% of cases occur just distal to the left subclavian artery. This is at the junction of the relatively fixed aortic arch and the more mobile descending aorta.

b) **False** The left main stem bronchus is displaced inferiorly.

c) **False** Up to 85% of patients die before reaching hospital.

d) **True** This is due to pressure on the oesophagus.

e) **True** Aortography only needs to be performed if there is a mediastinal haematoma. A completely normal CT effectively excludes the diagnosis.

31 a) True Bidirectional or reversal of flow within the portal vein, due to increased postsinusoidal pressure produced by hepatic venous obstruction, is typical.

b) **False** A characteristic 'spider web' pattern of intrahepatic venous collaterals is seen following a wedged hepatic venogram.

c) **True** The caudate lobe drains directly into the inferior vena cava (IVC) and, therefore, tends to hypertrophy in an attempt to take over the function of the liver.

d) **True** Obstruction of the suprahepatic IVC by a membranous web causing Budd–Chiari syndrome can successfully be treated with endoluminal stenting.

e) **True** There are also associations with other hypercoagulable states, such as polycythaemia, sickle cell disease, pregnancy and in patients receiving the contraceptive pill. Other causes include direct injury to the hepatic veins, tumour ingrowth and membranous obstruction to the suprahepatic IVC.

32 a) True Some practitioners use a mean pressure gradient of greater than 10 mm Hg.

b) **False** The 5-year patency rate with angioplasty alone is 70%–75%. This rises to 90%–95% following stenting.

c) **False** Stenting is only required if the distal blood flow is compromised.

d) **False** Stent failure is usually due to neointimal hyperplasia.

e) **True** These are called 'kissing stents', which avoid the problem of the proximal end of a single stent occluding the opposite common iliac artery.

33 a) True

b) **False**

c) **True**

d) **False**

e) **True**

34 a) **False** The IMA should be evaluated first so that the contrast-filled bladder does not obscure IMA branches.

b) **True** If a trial infusion of vasopressin controls the bleeding, then a prolonged infusion for 6–12 hours via the angiography catheter may avoid the need for surgery.

c) **True** Angiography is only used if endoscopy fails to control the bleeding.

d) **False** The IMA arises at the level of the L3 vertebral body.

e) **True** Diverticular haemorrhage accounts for approximately 60% of colonic bleeding. Angiodysplasia accounts for 20%, neoplasia 10% and colitis 5%–10%.

35 a) **False** This is seen in only 10%–20% of cases. It is often due to gastro-oesophageal reflux.

b) **True** Uncovered stents are less prone to this problem and are, therefore, preferred in the distal oesophagus.

c) **True** The procedure is usually performed under sedation with the patient on their right side and a suction catheter available to reduce the risk of aspiration

d) **False** There is no increase in the procedural morbidity following balloon rupture.

e) **False** Balloon dilatation is preferred for the treatment of achalasia. Multiple dilatations may be required. Metallic stents are usually avoided in benign disease.

36 a) **False** Colonic stents are typically used to decompress an obstructed bowel, allowing planned definitive surgery to be performed at a later stage.

b) **False** Uncovered stents are preferred, as they are associated with a lower risk of stent migration.

c) **False** Currently, the delivery systems are not long enough to place stents proximal to the descending colon.

d) **False** Although most commonly deployed for malignant disease, large-bowel obstruction secondary to diverticular disease can be treated with a colonic stent. This allows resection of the affected colon as a one-stage procedure at a later date.

e) **False**

37 a) **False** The combination of digital rectal examination and prostate specific antigen (PSA) is more sensitive than TRUS at detecting prostatic cancer.

b) **True** The prostate gland can be divided into three glandular zones (peripheral, central and transitional). The central and transitional zones are both heterogenous and hypoechogenic when compared to the more homogenous, echogenic peripheral zone.

c) **False** Prostatic cancer is normally hypoechoic (61% of cases) or isoechoic (35%) on ultrasound. Only rarely is it hyperechoic.

d) **True** In our practice, a single metronidazole suppository is combined with a single intravenous injection of gentamicin and a 5-day course of ciprofloxacin.

e) **False** At least six cores of tissue from all parts of the peripheral zone are necessary to sample the gland adequately.

38 a) **False** A dramatic bradycardia is often seen following closure of an arteriovenous fistula or a high-flow arteriovenous malformation (Branham's sign).

b) **False** Dissecting aneurysms of the ascending thoracic aorta require surgical treatment, whilst those of the descending aorta should be treated medically.

c) **True** These are due to cystic medial necrosis of the aortic wall.

d) **True** The left SVC usually drains into the coronary sinus.

e) **False** Histoplasmosis and tuberculosis are the most common causes of this condition.

39 a) **True** This makes them difficult to distinguish from vascular carcinomas on renal arteriograms. They may have a typical sunburst appearance.

b) **True** This is a recognised complication due to the spinal cord receiving its blood supply directly from the thoracic aorta.

c) **True** This is the most common complication of fibrosing mediastinitis, occurring in 60%–70% of cases.

d) **False** Nuclear medicine imaging using technetium-99m-labelled pertechnetate is the most sensitive method of detecting bleeding from a Meckel's diverticulum. Imaging every 5 minutes for a minimum of 1 hour is required.

e) **True** These are typically seen as well-defined, highly vascular masses.

40 a) **True** A multilobulated, 'beaded' appearance within the distal renal artery is typical of fibromuscular dysplasia and NF.

b) **False** About 75% of stenoses involve a short segment of the artery at the anastomosis site. About 25% involve a longer segment secondary to trauma during allograft harvesting or chronic rejection.

c) **True** The success of percutaneous transluminal angioplasty alone in treating ostial stenoses is not as great as for distal renal artery stenoses, often resulting in the need for stent placement.

d) **False** Renovascular disease accounts for less than 5% of cases of hypertension.

e) **True** A balloon should be inflated at the site of the extravasation and the patient transferred to the operating room for immediate surgical repair.

Chapter 11

Obstetrics and gynaecology

1   **Regarding ultrasonography in the first trimester of pregnancy, which of the following are true?**
    a)   Gestational sac volume is the most accurate estimate of gestational age in the first 8 weeks of pregnancy
    b)   The diameter of the yolk sac should not be more than 5 mm
    c)   The yolk sac is normally identified before the foetal pole
    d)   Cardiac pulsation becomes visible at the beginning of the eighth postmenstrual week
    e)   A normal intrauterine gestational sac and foetal pole exclude an ectopic pregnancy

2   **Which of the following statements are true?**
    a)   An empty gestational sac with a mean sac diameter of 10 mm and an elevated β human chorionic gonadotrophin (HCG) is consistent with a blighted ovum
    b)   β-HCG levels double every week in the first 8 weeks of pregnancy
    c)   An absent intrauterine pregnancy on ultrasonography and β-HCG levels between 1 000 and 2 000 IU is highly suspicious of an ectopic pregnancy
    d)   The risk of a second ectopic pregnancy is 10%
    e)   Vaginal bleeding is not usually associated with an ectopic pregnancy

3   **Regarding gestational trophoblastic disease, which of the following are true?**
    a)   Benign hydatidiform moles account for 60% of cases
    b)   On ultrasonography, multiple small intrauterine cysts with posterior acoustic enhancement are characteristic of hydatidiform moles
    c)   Large bilateral ovarian cysts are a frequent association
    d)   An invasive mole cannot be distinguished from a hydatidiform mole on ultrasonography
    e)   Choriocarcinoma follows a normal pregnancy in 1% of cases

4   **An axial ultrasonographic section through the foetal head for measurement of the biparietal diameter should include which of the following?**
    a)   The thalami
    b)   The cavum septum pellucidum
    c)   The third ventricle
    d)   A continuous echogenic midline
    e)   The cerebellum

5   **Regarding ultrasonography of the foetal head and neck, which of the following are true?**
    a)   About 50% of patients with a cleft lip and palate will have an associated congenital anomaly
    b)   Hypertelorism can be diagnosed on antenatal ultrasonography
    c)   Macroglossia cannot be diagnosed on ultrasonography
    d)   The lemon sign refers to the shape of the cerebellum in patients with hydrocephalus and spina bifida
    e)   The majority of cases of spina bifida also have Arnold–Chiari type II malformations

6   **Regarding the placenta, which of the following are true?**
    a) Ultrasonography should be performed with a full bladder in order to exclude placenta praevia
    b) The normal placenta should not measure more than 4 cm at its thickest point
    c) Painless vaginal bleeding is typical of placental abruption
    d) Placenta percreta refers to placental tissue invading through the myometrium at the site of a previous caesarean section
    e) An acute retroplacental bleed will appear echopoor on ultrasonography

7   **Causes of a raised maternal serum alpha-fetoprotein include which of the following?**
    a) Duodenal atresia
    b) Gastroschisis
    c) Meningocoele
    d) Omphalocoele
    e) Maternal hepatocellular carcinoma

8   **Which of the following statements are true?**
    a) Gadolinium diethylenetriaminepentaacetic acid (DTPA) chelate does not cross the placenta
    b) A foetal goitre can be distinguished from a cervical teratoma on magnetic resonance imaging (MRI)
    c) The most common posterolateral neck mass in the foetus is a cystic hygroma
    d) Premature rupture of membranes is the most common cause of oligohydramnios
    e) MRI is more accurate than ultrasound in diagnosing spina bifida

9   **Regarding endometriosis, which of the following are true?**
    a) About 30%–50% of women with endometriosis are infertile
    b) Endometriomas typically return coarse internal echoes on ultrasonography
    c) Endometriomas return a low signal on T1-weighted MRI
    d) Endometriosis within the chest usually presents with haemoptysis
    e) Endometriotic deposits of the gastrointestinal tract often erode through into the bowel lumen

10 **Which of the following statements are true?**
    a) Adenomyosis typically appears as areas of low echogenicity within the myometrium on transvaginal ultrasonography
    b) Cysts within the myometrium are commonly seen in patients with adenomyosis on transvaginal ultrasonography
    c) T1-weighted MRI best demonstrates normal uterine zonal anatomy
    d) Adenomyosis classically widens the outer myometrium on T2-weighted MRI
    e) Myometrial contractions can mimic adenomyosis

11 **Regarding uterine leiomyomas, which of the following are true?**
    a) They are typically of low T2 signal relative to the surrounding myometrium
    b) Cystic degeneration occurs in 30% of cases
    c) Red degeneration is associated with the contraceptive pill
    d) Calcification is usually peripheral
    e) Simple leiomyomas can metastasise

12 Which of the following statements are true regarding cervical carcinoma?
a) Invasion of the bladder represents stage IV disease
b) Cervical carcinoma is typically low signal on T2-weighted imaging
c) The inguinal region is the first site of metastatic lymph node involvement
d) Cervical carcinoma is typically isointense to the surrounding cervix on T1-weighted imaging
e) The vagina is isointense to striated muscle on all pulse sequences

13 Regarding perianal fistulae, which of the following are true?
a) The external anal sphincter is continuous with the levator ani
b) The internal sphincter can be divided without loss of continence
c) The internal and external anal sphincters cannot be separately resolved in normal patients on unenhanced MRI
d) If the ischioanal and ischiorectal fossae are involved on MRI, an intersphincteric abscess should be considered
e) About 70% of perianal fistulae are trans-sphincteric

14 Which of the following statements are true?
a) Gartner's duct cysts are typically located anterolateral to the upper two thirds of the vagina
b) Nabothian cysts occur in the posterolateral wall of the lower third of the vagina
c) The uterus is derived from the paired müllerian ducts
d) A unicornuate uterus is rarely associated with other anomalies
e) The risk of an ectopic pregnancy is higher in patients with a unicornuate uterus

15 Which of the following statements are true?
a) Intracavitary uterine polyps are associated with tamoxifen use
b) During the menstrual cycle, the endometrium should not measure more than 11 mm in thickness
c) The endometrium is echogenic relative to the surrounding myometrium throughout the menstrual cycle
d) The endometrium cannot be identified in the prepubertal female
e) The most common cause of postmenopausal bleeding is endometrial carcinoma

16 Which of the following statements are true?
a) A fluid collection within the endometrial cavity of a neonate is abnormal
b) Haematocolpos refers to a uterine cavity distended with blood
c) After puberty, the most common cause of haematocolpos is vaginal atresia
d) Congenital haematometrocolpos is usually associated with other anomalies
e) Haematometra is a cause of ureteric obstruction

17 Regarding mature cystic teratomas of the ovary (dermoid cysts), which of the following are true?
a) They typically present before 10 years of age
b) They are typically multilocular on ultrasonography
c) Ectodermal tissue is invariably present
d) The presence of fat on MRI confirms the diagnosis
e) Malignant degeneration occurs in 1%–3% of cases

18 Regarding polycystic ovaries, which of the following are true?

a) The ovaries are enlarged on ultrasonography in 95% of cases
b) There is a decrease in the ratio of luteinising hormone to follicular stimulating hormone
c) There is an increased risk of endometrial carcinoma
d) Cysts of 5–8 mm are characteristically present throughout the ovary
e) They are seen in patients with trophoblastic disease

19 Regarding foetal anomalies, which of the following are true?

a) The triple screen for Down's syndrome refers to the combination of maternal alpha-fetoprotein, oestriol and HCG levels
b) Short femur and humerus lengths are indicators of Down's syndrome
c) The nuchal-fold thickness is most prominent between 11 and 13 weeks
d) Endocardial cushion defects are strongly associated with Down's syndrome
e) Separation of the big toe from the remaining toes is a strong sign of Down's syndrome

20 Regarding ovarian tumours, which of the following are true?

a) Sex cord stromal tumours constitute 80%–90% of malignant ovarian tumours
b) Ovarian fibromas are typically high signal on T2-weighted imaging
c) Sex cord stromal tumours typically cause pseudomyxoma peritonei
d) Epithelial ovarian neoplasms often produce androgens or oestrogens
e) Granulosa cell tumours spread early to peritoneal surfaces

Answers

1 a) **False**   Once the foetus can be identified (5–6 weeks), then the crown-to-rump length becomes the most accurate measurement. The biparietal diameter becomes the most accurate towards the end of the first trimester.

  b) **True**   A large yolk sac (greater than 5 mm) is highly suggestive of an abnormal pregnancy and embryonic death.

  c) **True**   The yolk sac can be identified on transvaginal scanning at 4–5 weeks. The foetal pole is visualised at 5–6 weeks. The yolk sac is the first structure identified within a normal gestational sac.

  d) **False**   Cardiac pulsation is identified almost as soon as the foetal pole is visualised. This is usually at the beginning of the sixth postmenstrual week on transabdominal scanning.

  e) **False**   A coexisting intrauterine and ectopic pregnancy (heterotopic pregnancy) is extremely rare in spontaneous conceptions (1 in 30 000 pregnancies), but it is increasingly seen in patients undergoing assisted conception (up to 1 in 2 000 pregnancies).

2 a) **True**   A 'blighted ovum' (anembryonic pregnancy) still produces β-HCG due to production by trophoblasts in the wall of the gestational sac.

  b) **False**   Levels of β-HCG double every 2–3 days in the first 8 weeks of pregnancy.

  c) **True**   This is true even if an adnexal mass cannot be identified.

  d) **False**   The risk of a second ectopic pregnancy is 25%. Other risk factors include: previous tubal surgery, previous pelvic inflammatory disease, endometriosis, induced ovulation, an intrauterine contraceptive device *in situ* and salpingitis isthmica nodosa.

  e) **False**   Vaginal bleeding is present in 75%–85% of ectopic pregnancies.

3 a) **False**   This benign form accounts for 80%–90% of cases. An invasive mole is seen in 5%–8% of cases and choriocarcinoma in 1%–2% of cases.

  b) **True**   However, this typical appearance is often not seen until the second trimester.

  c) **True**   Multiple theca-lutein cysts, stimulated by the elevated levels of β-HCG, occur in up to 50% of cases. These may take up to 4 months to regress.

  d) **False**   Invasive moles form pockets of trophoblastic cells within the myometrium. These are highly vascular and are often identified on colour Doppler scanning.

  e) **False**   About 20%–25% of choriocarcinomas follow a normal pregnancy. About 50% follow a previous hydatidiform mole.

4 a) **True**
  b) **True**
  c) **True**
  d) **False**
  e) **False**

   The biparietal diameter is used for estimating the gestational age after 12 weeks. Its accuracy declines after 28 weeks, at which time it should be combined with a second measurement, such as femur length. Measurements are made from the outer side of the near skull to the inner side of the distal skull.

5 a) **True** There is a particularly strong association with trisomy syndromes 13 and 18. Typically these are paramedian clefts. A median cleft lip is much rarer and may be associated with intracranial abnormalities, such as holoprosencephaly.

b) **True** Causes include craniosynostoses, cleft lip and palate, frontal encephalocoeles and exposure to teratogens, such as phenytoin.

c) **False** When the tongue is enlarged it persistently protrudes from the open mouth. Intermittent protrusion is often seen in normal foetuses. It is an important observation because of its association with Beckwith–Wiedemann syndrome.

d) **False** The lemon sign refers to the shape of the head in patients with hydrocephalus and spina bifida. Typically the head is pointed anteriorly on the transverse section.

e) **True** In Arnold–Chiari type II malformation, the cerebellar vermis herniates into the foramen magnum. There is displacement of the fourth ventricle and obstructive hydrocephalus. The cerebellum is typically bowed posteriorly, resulting in the banana sign.

6 a) **False** A full bladder causing the internal os to appear covered by the placenta may artificially lengthen the cervix.

b) **True** A thick placenta can be a sign of uncontrolled maternal diabetes, intrauterine infections or hydrops foetalis.

c) **False** Painless vaginal bleeding is typical of placenta praevia. Bleeding is often painful with placental abruption.

d) **True** Placenta accreta implies that the chorionic villi are in direct contact with the myometrium. In placenta increta the villi invade the myometrium. In placenta percreta invasion extends through the uterine wall. All types can cause persistent postpartum haemorrhage.

e) **False** Initially the blood may be hyperechoic or isoechoic. This can make differentiation from the adjacent placenta very difficult. The haematoma will become hypoechoic within 2 weeks.

7 **All true** Alpha-fetoprotein is produced by the yolk sac and the immature foetal liver. It is classically raised in open neural tube defects. Other foetal causes include: ventral wall defects, upper gastrointestinal obstruction, cystic hygroma, teratoma, amniotic band syndrome and feto-maternal haemorrhage.

8 a) **False** Hence, its use in pregnancy is avoided. There are no known deleterious effects of MRI on the foetus, but it is generally avoided in the first trimester when organogenesis occurs.

b) **True** A foetal goitre is usually secondary to maternal thyroid disease. On a T1-weighted fast spin echo sequence, a goitre returns a high signal when compared with other anterior neck masses in the foetus (teratoma, haemangioma).

c) **True** This is a fluid-filled lymphatic malformation, which is associated with Turner's syndrome, trisomies 13, 18 and 21, Noonan's syndrome and foetal alcohol syndrome.

d) **True** Other causes include renal anomalies, posterior urethral valves and growth retardation. MRI can be useful, particularly to clarify renal anomalies when the oligohydramnios makes ultrasonography difficult.

e) **False** Ultrasound has much greater spatial resolution than MRI.

9 a) **True** In addition, 20% of infertile women have endometriosis. Infertility may relate to autoimmune factors as well as anatomical abnormalities.

b) **False** A homogenous, hypoechoic cyst with diffuse low-level internal echoes is the characteristic ultrasonographic appearance. Atypical examples may be anechoic and they may be unilocular or multilocular.

c) **False** Endometriomas are typically high signal on T1-weighted imaging. This is due to blood breakdown products within the cyst. The appearances are particularly striking on T1-weighted imaging following fat saturation. This sequence helps distinguish a dermoid cyst (low signal) from an endometrioma (high signal).

d) **False** More than 70% of cases present with a pneumothorax. This may be recurrent, presenting at menstruation. A small number of patients present with haemoptysis or a haemothorax.

e) **False** Deposits are serosal and erode through the subserosal layers causing thickening of the muscularis propria. The underlying mucosa is almost never breeched. The inferior surface of the sigmoid colon and the anterior surface of the rectum are the most common sites. The gastrointestinal tract is involved in 10%–30% of cases.

10 a) **True** Adenomyosis refers to the presence of heterotopic endometrial glands within the myometrium, with associated smooth muscle hyperplasia. More than 75% of patients show areas of low echogenicity or heterogeneity on transvaginal ultrasonography.

b) **True** Cysts are present in 50% of cases and represent dilated cystic glands or haemorrhagic areas within the abnormal myometrium. They are usually less than 5 mm in diameter.

c) **False** T2-weighted MRI demonstrates normal zonal anatomy better than T1-weighted MRI or T1-weighted MRI with contrast enhancement. On T2-weighted imaging the endometrium is high signal, the junctional zone or inner myometrium is low signal and the outer myometrium is of intermediate signal. The sagittal plane usually provides the best demonstration of uterine zonal anatomy.

d) **False** Adenomyosis is predominantly low signal on T2-weighted MRI. This gives the appearance of a widened low signal junctional zone. A junctional zone greater than 12 mm in diameter is highly specific for adenomyosis.

e) **True** Myometrial contractions can thicken the junctional zone and, therefore, mimic adenomyosis. Adenomyosis itself can mimic endometrial carcinoma or alter the staging accuracy of endometrial carcinoma.

11 a) **True** This is due to hyalinisation and is present in 60% of uterine leiomyomas. Intermediate signal on T1-weighted images is also typical.

b) **False** Cystic degeneration is rare and occurs in approximately 4% of cases.

c) **True** Both pregnancy and the contraceptive pill are associated with red degeneration. Usually there is obstruction of the peripheral draining veins resulting in haemorrhagic infarction.

d) **False** However, red degeneration may result in peripheral calcification. Typically the appearance is of scattered, amorphous calcification marking the site of hyaline degeneration.

e) **True** Rarely, there is direct growth into local veins followed by distant metastases (benign metastasising leiomyoma). Dissemination throughout the peritoneal cavity is also recognised.

12 a) **True**   Stage I disease is carcinoma confined to the cervix. Stage II is tumour extending beyond the uterus, but not to the pelvic sidewall or the lower third of the vagina. Stage III is tumour extending to the pelvic sidewall or to the lower third of the vagina. Stage IV is invasion of the bladder or rectal mucosa (IV-A) or distant metastases (IV-B).

   b) **False**   Cervical carcinoma is usually of intermediate signal relative to the surrounding low signal cervical stroma on T2-weighted imaging.

   c) **False**   Lymph node spread is typically to the iliac and then periaortic nodal groups.

   d) **True**   Most tumours are best identified on T2-weighted imaging. Small tumours, however, are most conspicuous on T1-weighted sequences after contrast enhancement.

   e) **True**   The vaginal vault may be high signal on T2-weighted imaging due to vaginal secretions.

13 a) **True**   The internal anal sphincter is continuous with the circular smooth muscle of the rectum.

   b) **True**   Although the internal sphincter accounts for 85% of resting anal tone, it is the external sphincter that is important for continence.

   c) **True**   Anal endosonography demonstrates the sphincter mechanism and intersphincteric plane, but shows the external sphincter less reliably. It may not identify abscesses lying some distance from the probe and may not distinguish fibrosis from infection. MRI is superior in this regard.

   d) **False**   This implies the presence of a trans-sphincteric fistula/abscess or translevator disease.

   e) **False**   About 70% of perianal fistulae are intersphincteric and 20% are trans-sphincteric. Extrasphincteric and supralevator fistulae are rare. The fistula starts as an infection in the anal mucosal gland. The chronic sepsis spreads to the intersphincteric plane (cryptoglandular hypothesis) from where it may track in the intersphincteric plane (intersphincteric fistula), through the external sphincter or above the levator muscle (supralevator). These may be associated with abscesses anywhere along their length.

14 a) **True**   Gartner's duct cysts occur in 1%–2% of females and develop in remnants of the wolffian duct system. Although they are incidental findings, they may be associated with renal tract anomalies.

   b) **False**   This describes a Bartholin's cyst. Mucous retention within endocervical glands is termed a nabothian cyst. Gartner's, Bartholin's and nabothian cysts are all high signal on T2-weighted MRI.

   c) **True**   The müllerian ducts form the uterus, the Fallopian tubes and the upper two thirds of the vagina. The ovaries are formed from primitive germ cells and the lower third of the vagina arises from the vaginal plate.

   d) **False**   About 40% of patients with a unicornuate uterus have associated renal or ureteric abnormalities. These include renal agenesis, ectopia, fusion, malrotation and duplication.

   e) **True**   About 25% of patients with uterine abnormalities have fertility problems.

15 a) **True** About 60% of women receiving long-term tamoxifen will develop changes in the endometrial cavity. These may be multiple polyps or cystic and echogenic areas due to subendometrial adenomyosis. There is also a small increased risk of endometrial carcinoma.

b) **False** During the early proliferative stage, the endometrium becomes echogenic and measures 5–7 mm. In the late proliferative stage, the endometrium becomes hypoechoic with an echogenic basal layer and can measure up to 11 mm in thickness. During the secretory phase, the endometrium again becomes echogenic and can measure up to 16 mm in thickness.

c) **False** See b).

d) **False** The endometrium is seen as a thin echogenic line in the prepubertal female.

e) **False** About 75% of cases of postmenopausal bleeding are due to endometrial atrophy. Endometrial cancer is responsible in 10% of cases. Other causes include polyps, submucosal fibroids, endometrial hyperplasia and oestrogen withdrawal.

16 a) **False** Approximately 25% of normal neonates have a small fluid collection within the uterine cavity. The uterus is typically tubular at birth with the cervix and uterine body being similar in size.

b) **False** Haematocolpos refers to the vagina distended with blood and haematometra to the uterine cavity distended with blood. Mayer–Rokitansky–Küster–Hauser syndrome refers to agenesis of the vagina with intact ovaries/Fallopian tubes and variable anomalies of the uterus and urinary tract.

c) **False** An imperforate hymen is the most common cause of haematocolpos. Other causes include a transverse vaginal septum and vaginal atresia.

d) **True** Other associations include imperforate anus, renal agenesis, sacral atresia and oesophageal atresia.

e) **True** The ureters typically become compressed as they pass anteriorly at the level of the cervix.

17 a) **False** The mean age at presentation is 30 years. They are however the most common paediatric ovarian tumour. Immature teratomas typically present in the first two decades of life.

b) **False** About 88% are unilocular. Classically, there is a raised nodule extending into the lumen of the cyst. This is called a Rokitansky nodule. Any hair within the cyst arises from this nodule.

c) **True** These tumours contain material from at least two of the three germ cell layers. Ectoderm is always present. Mesoderm and endoderm are present in the majority of cases.

d) **True** Hence, MRI with chemical shift imaging and fat-saturation techniques is important.

e) **True** Surgery is usually performed to avoid torsion or cyst rupture.

18 a) **False**   About 70% of cases have bilaterally enlarged ovaries (greater than 14 cm³).
In 30% of cases, the ovaries are of normal size.

b) **False**   The reverse is true. The condition is caused by decreased conversion of androgen to oestrogen. This results in immature follicles that do not develop into graafian follicles.

c) **True**   This is due to chronic non-cyclical oestrogen stimulation.

d) **False**   The cysts are typically subcapsular. The central stroma of the ovary is of increased echogenicity. In 25% of cases, the ovaries are hypoechoic without demonstrable follicles.

e) **False**   Trophoblastic disease typically causes hyperstimulation of the ovaries with large multiseptated cysts secondary to elevated HCG levels. There may also be ascites and severe electrolyte imbalance. Polycystic ovaries may be seen in congenital adrenal hyperplasia.

19 a) **True**   If all three levels are elevated, the risk of Down's syndrome is increased.

b) **True**   If the humerus and femur are less than 91% of the expected length for gestational age, there is an increased risk of Down's syndrome.

c) **True**   A measurement of greater than 6 mm at this time is a strong indicator of Down's syndrome.

d) **True**   Endocardial cushion defects are seen in 25% of cases of Down's syndrome. Other thoracic anomalies in Down's syndrome include membranous ventricular septal defects, ostium primum atrial septal defects, cleft mitral valve, patent ductus arteriosus, 11 rib pairs (in 25% of cases) and a hypersegmented manubrium (in 90%).

e) **False**   This is termed a sandal toe. It is a weak sign of Down's syndrome.

20 a) **False**   Ovarian tumours are classified as epithelial, germ cell or stromal/sex cord tumours. Epithelial tumours constitute two thirds of all ovarian tumours and 80%–90% of malignant ovarian neoplasms.

b) **False**   Ovarian fibromas account for 4% of ovarian neoplasms. They are benign tumours that may be associated with ascites and pleural effusions (Meigs' syndrome). On T2-weighted MRI they are very low signal, although scattered areas of high signal representing oedema can often be seen.

c) **False**   Pseudomyxoma peritonei is typically caused by mucinous cystadenocarcinoma of the appendix or ovary.

d) **False**   Hormone production is typical of the sex cord stromal tumours. Epithelial tumours rarely produce hormones.

e) **False**   About 90% of granulosa cell tumours are confined to the ovary at presentation (stage 1). They are predominantly solid tumours with multiple cystic spaces, which frequently produce oestrogens and more rarely androgens.

Chapter 12

Nuclear medicine and positron emission tomography imaging

1   Which of the following are true regarding the physics of nuclear medicine?
   a)   Isomers are defined as nuclides with the same number of protons
   b)   One becquerel (Bq) indicates one radioactive disintegration per second
   c)   The biological half-life of a radioisotope is usually less than the effective half-life
   d) ^{99m}Tc emits γ rays with energy of 140 keV
   e)   Single photon emission computed tomography (SPECT) has a better spatial resolution than conventional planar imaging

2   Regarding the design and function of a gamma camera, which of the following are true?
   a)   The collimator lies between the crystal and the photomultiplier tubes
   b)   The normal camera crystal is made of Tl-activated sodium iodide
   c)   The photomultiplier tubes convert electrical energy into light photons
   d)   The energy of the Compton tail lies above that of the photopeak
   e)   Intrinsic resolution is always better than system resolution

3   Which of the following are true of positron emission tomography (PET)?
   a)   It utilises a process known as annihilation coincidence
   b)   It normally requires close proximity to a cyclotron
   c)   PET images have a higher spatial resolution than SPECT images
   d)   On PET scans using 2-[^{18}F]-fluoro-2-deoxy-D-glucose (^{18}FDG), most tumours appear as focal 'cold' spots
   e)   The sensitivity of ^{18}FDG scanning is less in diabetic patients

4   Regarding ^{99m}technetium (^{99m}Tc) methylene diphosphonate (MDP) bone scans, which of the following are true?
   a)   MDP is absorbed onto hydroxyapatite crystals in bone
   b)   More than 70% of ^{99m}Tc MDP is renally excreted in the first 24 hours postinjection
   c)   The static images are routinely obtained 4–6 hours post-injection
   d) ^{99m}Tc MDP is normally taken up by the salivary glands
   e) ^{99m}Tc MDP cardiac uptake is seen in unstable angina pectoris

5   Which of the following are classically 'hot' on a ^{99m}Tc MDP bone scan?
   a)   Acute fracture within 12 hours of injury
   b)   Bone island
   c)   Fibrous dysplasia
   d)   Reflex sympathetic dystrophy
   e)   Multiple myeloma

6   Which of the following can cause a 'superscan' appearance on a ^{99m}Tc MDP bone scan?
   a)   Mastocytosis
   b)   Osteomalacia
   c)   Bony lymphoma
   d)   Hyperthyroidism
   e)   Fibrous dysplasia

7   **Which of the following are true of scintigraphy and bony neoplasia?**
   a) An increase in activity around metastases can indicate a response to therapy
   b) Osteoid osteomas are classically 'hot' with a central 'cold' nidus
   c) In 5% of bone scans negative for metastases, the radiograph will be positive
   d) Radiotherapy usually leads to a well-defined 'hot' area, which may mask a deposit
   e) In a patient with a known malignancy, 40%–50% of solitary 'hot' spots are malignant

8   **Regarding the scintigraphic assessment of a joint prosthesis, which of the following are true?**
   a) Increased MDP activity over the greater trochanter is diagnostic of an inflammatory bursitis
   b) A normal, noncemented total hip replacement (THR) will be 'hot' 12 months after surgery
   c) A 'hot' knee prosthesis 18 months after surgery is abnormal
   d) Prosthetic loosening results in a scan that is 'hot' on blood pool and delayed phases
   e) Uptake of ^{67}gallium (^{67}Ga) around a THR that is more than 2 years old suggests infection

9   **Regarding bone marrow imaging, which of the following are true?**
   a) Only 10% of an injected ^{99m}Tc sulphur colloid dose is taken up by bone marrow
   b) A bony metastasis classically shows as a 'hot spot' on a marrow scan
   c) In normal adults, activity should not be seen in femora
   d) Appendicular extension of bone marrow activity can be seen in myelofibrosis
   e) Reduced central marrow activity is seen in aplastic anaemia

10 **Concerning the radiopharmaceuticals used in lung scintigraphy, which of the following are true?**
   a) ^{99m}Tc macroaggregated albumin (MAA) particles should be greater than 10 μm in size
   b) A right-to-left shunt is an absolute contraindication to the use of ^{99m}Tc MAA
   c) If ^{133}xenon (^{133}Xe) is used as the ventilation agent, a perfusion scan should be performed first
   d) ^{81m}Krypton has a half-life of about 13 seconds
   e) About 10% of administered ^{99m}Tc diethylenetriaminepenta-acetic acid (DTPA) aerosol reaches the lung parenchyma

11 **Regarding scintigraphy for suspected pulmonary emboli, which of the following are true?**
   a) There is normally more activity posteriorly than anteriorly on perfusion images
   b) Costophrenic angles are better seen on ^{133}Xe ventilation images than on MAA images
   c) The presence of the stripe sign makes a pulmonary embolus in that region unlikely
   d) If ventilation in more than 75% of the lung is abnormal, the study is indeterminate for pulmonary emboli
   e) Pulmonary emboli typically appear as reversed mismatched defects

12 **Which of the following are causes of total loss of perfusion to one lung on a ventilation/perfusion (V/Q) scan?**
   a) Swyer–James (Macleod's) syndrome
   b) A Blalock–Taussig shunt
   c) Pleural effusion
   d) Pneumothorax
   e) Histoplasmosis

13 **Regarding the radionuclides used in cardiac imaging, which of the following are true?**
   a) Cellular uptake of ^{201}thallium (^{201}Tl) chloride relies on an intact Na$^+$/K$^+$ ATPase pump
   b) ^{201}Tl chloride has a physical half-life of 73 hours
   c) ^{99m}Tc sestamibi is preferred over ^{201}Tl chloride for obese patients
   d) ^{99m}Tc sestamibi, unlike ^{201}Tl, undergoes no significant redistribution phase
   e) ^{99m}Tc teboroxime has a biological half-life of 10–20 minutes

14 **Which of the following are true of stress testing in cardiac scintigraphy?**
   a) Prior to a treadmill test, patients are routinely fasted
   b) The typical target heart rate in a treadmill test is 220 minus the patient's age in years
   c) Failure to achieve target heart rate in an exercise test reduces sensitivity for ischaemia by 50%
   d) The normal lung:heart activity ratio is less than 0.5
   e) Adenosine is the agent of choice for pharmacological stress testing in patients with asthma

15 **Which of the following typically cause a reduction in myocardial uptake of ^{201}Tl?**
   a) Hibernating myocardium
   b) Cardiac sarcoidosis
   c) Cardiac amyloidosis
   d) Left bundle branch block
   e) Mitral valve prolapse

16 **Which of the following are true of cardiac PET studies?**
   a) Exercise stress testing is usually preferred over pharmacological stress testing
   b) ^{82}Rubidium (^{82}Rb) is used to demonstrate cardiac perfusion
   c) Ischaemic myocardium is typically 'cold' on an ^{18}FDG PET study
   d) Hibernating myocardium cannot be identified by cardiac PET studies
   e) Decreased perfusion and metabolism indicate infarcted myocardium

17 **Which of the following are true of ventricular function studies?**
   a) First-pass studies are usually performed with ^{99m}Tc-labelled red cells
   b) Left-to-right cardiac shunts can be detected on first-pass studies
   c) Wall movement is optimally assessed with gated blood-pool studies
   d) The normal value for left ventricular ejection fraction (LVEF) is 50%–65%
   e) The LVEF normally falls slightly after commencing exercise

18 **Concerning the radioisotopes utilised in renal imaging, which of the following are true?**
   a) ^{99m}Tc mercaptoacetyltriglycine (MAG$_3$) is mostly cleared by glomerular filtration
   b) ^{99m}Tc MAG$_3$ is the radionuclide of choice in renal insufficiency
   c) ^{99m}Tc DTPA is mostly cleared by glomerular filtration
   d) Dimercaptosuccinic acid (DMSA) is the agent of choice for calculating renal function in the presence of an obstruction
   e) After 3 hours, 50% of a ^{99m}Tc DMSA dose accumulates in renal tubular cells

19 **Which of the following are true regarding a normal renal scintigram?**
   a) On perfusion images, peak renal activity occurs 3–6 seconds after peak aortic activity
   b) Peak cortical activity occurs 3–5 minutes postinjection
   c) Peak renal activity should be equal or higher than peak spleen activity
   d) Quantitative split renal function is estimated between 5–10 minutes postinjection
   e) Visualisation of a ureter on a MAG$_3$ study is abnormal

20 **Which of the following are true of angiotensin-converting enzyme (ACE) inhibition renography?**
   a) ACE inhibitors predominantly exert their effect on the afferent arteriole
   b) Diuretics should be withheld for 48 hours before an ACE inhibitor renogram
   c) Unilaterally reduced renal perfusion is diagnostic of renal artery stenosis (RAS)
   d) This test is particularly suited to detecting bilateral stenoses
   e) A 10% fall in 20-minute cortical activity on an MAG_3 renogram indicates renal artery stenosis

21 **Concerning vesico-ureteric reflux radioisotope studies, which of the following are true?**
   a) The radiation dose of radionuclide cystography is lower than that of fluoroscopic cystography
   b) Vesico-ureteric reflux occurs only during the bladder-filling phase in 20% of cases
   c) On serial studies, the threshold volume required for reflux decreases
   d) Isotope studies do not allow grading of reflux as accurately as fluoroscopy
   e) Vesico-ureteric reflux in a 4-year-old with a normal DMSA scan does not warrant the use of antibiotics

22 **Regarding the scintigraphic assessment of renal transplants, which of the following are true?**
   a) Typically acute tubular necrosis results in normal renal perfusion, but decreased excretion
   b) Acute rejection is typified by reduced renal perfusion and excretion
   c) Early visualisation of the inferior vena cava is typical of an arteriovenous fistula
   d) Failure to visualise an isotope outside the collecting system excludes a urinoma
   e) Haematoma and urinomas cannot be distinguished by scintigraphy

23 **Which of the following are true regarding gastric emptying studies?**
   a) Liquids are more sensitive than solids in detecting abnormal gastric emptying
   b) After a solid meal, there is an exponential clearance of activity from the stomach
   c) The emptying half-time of the normal stomach is usually 30 minutes for liquids
   d) Anorexia nervosa typically results in rapid gastric emptying
   e) Thyrotoxicosis typically causes rapid gastric emptying

24 **Concerning Meckel's diverticulum scanning, which of the following are true?**
   a) The sensitivity of pertechnetate scintigraphy falls after adolescence
   b) Activity in a diverticulum usually appears 1–2 hours postinjection
   c) Glucagon administration results in an increased uptake of pertechnetate
   d) A tubular area of increased activity in the right iliac fossa is typical of a Meckel's diverticulum
   e) Barrett's oesophagus can produce a false positive scan

25 **Which of the following are true of radionuclide tests and gastrointestinal (GI) bleeding?**
   a) Radionuclide tests are usually more sensitive for GI bleeding than angiography
   b) ^{99m}Tc-labelled red cells have a longer half-life than ^{99m}Tc sulphur colloid
   c) ^{99m}Tc sulphur colloid is more sensitive for bleeding in the upper than the lower GI tract
   d) Uptake in the bowel that does not alter in location or intensity is typical for GI bleeding
   e) The specificity of isotope studies is decreased in Osler–Weber–Rendu syndrome

26 **Concerning imaging with ^{99m}Tc-labelled iminodiacetic acid (IDA) agents, which of the following are true?**
   a) Of the injected ^{99m}Tc-labelled IDA, 85%–99% is excreted into the bile
   b) On a normal study, the gallbladder is visualised within 1 hour of injection
   c) Normally, the gallbladder is visualised before the duodenum
   d) Morphine can usefully be administered during the study in order to contract the gallbladder
   e) The width of activity in the common bile duct correlates closely with actual diameter

27 **Which of the following are true of biliary studies?**
   a) Alcoholism is a recognised cause of failure to visualise the gallbladder 4 hours postinjection
   b) The rim sign refers to the appearance of activity in the hypervascular gallbladder wall
   c) In 4% of cases of acute cholecystitis, the gallbladder is seen to fill on delayed images
   d) The presence of a duodenal diverticulum lowers test sensitivity for cholecystitis
   e) Chronic cholecystitis and acalculous cholecystitis can be differentiated

28 **Concerning paediatric and postoperative cholescintigraphy, which of the following are true?**
   a) Neonatal liver immaturity prevents biliary atresia studies in the first 2 months of life
   b) Concurrent phenobarbitone administration hinders paediatric biliary atresia studies
   c) On a normal paediatric dimethyl hepato-iminodiacetic acid (HIDA) study, the liver is visualised 5 minutes after injection
   d) Choledochal and pancreatic cysts can be differentiated on cholescintigraphy
   e) Cholescintigraphy is more specific than ultrasonography for postoperative bile leaks

29 **Regarding the radionuclides used in thyroid studies, which of the following are true?**
   a) ^{123}Iodine (^{123}I) is the isotope of choice for routine diagnostic imaging
   b) ^{123}I is usually administered by intravenous injection
   c) ^{99m}Tc pertechnetate is trapped, but not organified, by the thyroid
   d) ^{131}I has a half-life of 8 days
   e) ^{131}I is the isotope of choice for demonstrating retrosternal thyroid tissue

30 **Which of the following are true of thyroid nodule imaging?**
   a) About 10% of 'hot' nodules are malignant
   b) About 80%–90% of 'cold' nodules are benign
   c) About 25% of 'hot' nodules are palpable
   d) Less than 5% of dominant nodules in a multinodular goitre are malignant
   e) A classical discordant nodule is ^{99m}Tc pertechnetate 'hot' and ^{123}I 'cold'

31 **Regarding thyroid scintigraphy and uptake studies, which of the following are true?**
   a) Decreased ^{123}I uptake is seen in hypoalbuminaemia
   b) Increased ^{123}I uptake is seen in thyroiditis
   c) Low tracer uptake almost never occurs in hyperthyroidism
   d) A 'hot' nodule with central photopenia has the same malignant risk as a 'cold' nodule
   e) A rise in thyroglobulin levels after ^{131}I ablation suggests thyroid cancer recurrence

32 **Which of the following are true regarding parathyroid scintigraphy?**
  a) ^{201}Tl is utilised in subtraction imaging, as it localises to the parathyroid glands only
  b) With ^{201}Tl/^{99m}Tc pertechnetate subtraction imaging, lesion specificity is only 40%
  c) Parathyroid scintigraphy is more sensitive to adenomas than gland hyperplasia
  d) On delayed ^{99m}Tc sestamibi scans, parathyroid adenomas typically remain 'hot'
  e) ^{99m}Tc sestamibi has a half-life of 6 hours

33 **Which of the following are true regarding ^{99m}TC hexamethylpropyleneamineoxime (HMPAO) brain studies?**
  a) ^{99m}Tc HMPAO does not readily cross the normal blood–brain barrier
  b) White matter takes up the agent more readily than grey matter
  c) There is reduced uptake in the basal ganglia (caudate) in Huntington's chorea
  d) In Alzheimer's disease, there is a reduction in the cortical/cerebellar uptake ratio
  e) Interictal scans will typically show decreased uptake in the seizure focus

34 **Concerning ^{67}gallium (^{67}Ga) scintigraphy, which of the following are true?**
  a) There is improved lesion detection in patients with haemochromatosis
  b) Neutropenia is a recognised cause of a false negative scan
  c) Uptake in the lacrimal glands is not normal
  d) Faint activity in the kidneys is normal up to 96 hours postinjection
  e) It has a physical half-life of 78 hours

35 **Which of the following chest conditions take up ^{67}Ga citrate avidly?**
  a) Kaposi's sarcoma
  b) *Pneumocystis carinii* pneumonia
  c) Lymphoma
  d) Bacterial pneumonia
  e) Sarcoidosis

36 **Which of the following are true of labelled white cell scanning?**
  a) The white cells are most commonly labelled with ^{111}indium (^{111}In) oxine
  b) ^{111}In oxine-labelled white cell studies are superior to ^{67}Ga for abdominal imaging
  c) On a normal ^{111}In oxine scan, activity is greater in the spleen than the liver
  d) Visualisation of the lungs on a 4-hour image suggests thoracic pathology
  e) The white cells that are labelled must originate from the patient

37 **Which of the following are true of studies using labelled white cells?**
  a) Isotope uptake around a surgical drainage tube indicates a residual abscess
  b) White cell studies are more sensitive to chronic infection than an acute process
  c) Crohn's disease is typically 'cold' on an ^{111}In oxine-labelled white cell study
  d) Uncomplicated congestive cardiac failure is typically 'hot' on a white cell study
  e) The sensitivity of white cell studies falls significantly if the patient is receiving antibiotics

38 **Which of the following tumours are 'hot' on a metaiodobenzylguanidine (MIBG) scan?**
  a) Ganglioneuroma
  b) Extra-adrenal phaeochromocytoma
  c) Medullary thyroid carcinoma
  d) Neuroblastoma
  e) Carcinoid tumour

39 Which of the following are 'hot' on a ^{111}In octreotide study?

a) Neuroblastoma

b) Gastrinoma

c) Sarcoidosis

d) Breast cancer

e) Kidneys

40 Which of the following are true?

a) Focal nodular hyperplasia is classically 'cold' on a ^{99m}Tc sulphur colloid study

b) The 'nubbin' sign is consistent with testicular torsion

c) Lymphoscintigraphy is contraindicated in congenital lymphoedema

d) On cisternography, activity is usually seen in the basal cistern after 2–4 hours

e) No ventricular activity on cisternography suggests normal pressure hydrocephalus

Answers

1 a) **False**   This is the definition of isotopes (e.g. [131]iodine [I] and ^{125}I). Isomers are defined as nuclides with the same number of protons and neutrons, but with a different energy state (e.g. [99]Tc and ^{99m}Tc). Isomers (radionuclides) may be unstable and are denoted by the symbol 'm' for metastable if the excited state has a fairly long half-life. They become stable by emitting energy (a process known as isomeric transition); their detection is useful in nuclear medicine.

     b) **True**   This is the SI unit of radioactivity. One megabecquerel (MBq) equals one million disintegrations per second. The amount of radioactive agent given during a study is recorded in becquerels (e.g. 500 MBq for a bone scan).

     c) **False**   The effective half-life (t_{eff}) is shorter than the biological (t_{bio}) and physical (t_{phys}) half-lives. A radionuclide undergoes a gradual reduction in activity (physical half-life), but at the same time is being eliminated by the body (biological half-life ($1/t_{eff} = 1/t_{phys} + 1/t_{biol}$). Effective half-life varies from person to person.

     d) **True**   [99m]Tc is the most commonly used isotope for various reasons: it emits rays with enough energy to exit the patient's body, but not so much that they will not be absorbed by the camera; it has a physical half-life of 6 hours; it decays by pure gamma emission; it can be easily produced from [99]molybdenum (Mo) in a generator; and it can be readily attached to a wide variety of compounds, such as dimercaptosuccinic acid (DMSA) and methylene diphosphonate (MDP).

     e) **False**   As the parallel hole collimator rotates around the patient (in order to obtain cross-sectional images), far fewer counts are obtained per position than in static imaging. Therefore, noise levels are high. To reduce this, a matrix with large pixels is used, which worsens the spatial resolution.

2 a) **False** A lead collimator, containing multiple small holes (approximately 20 000), lies between the patient and the crystal. This is used to localise the activity coming from the patient to a specific location. Only gamma rays travelling parallel to holes can reach the camera, thus locating any radioactive source along its line of sight; rays travelling obliquely are absorbed.

b) **True** This is used because it has a high atomic number (53) and will absorb most (90%) of the ^{99m}Tc gamma rays. It is temperature sensitive and hygroscopic. Thus, it needs a protective shield, which is usually made of aluminium.

c) **False** The photomultiplier tubes absorb light photons coming off the crystal and convert them into electrons, which, via a system of dinodes, are accelerated towards an anode where they produce a voltage that can be measured. Thus, the photomultiplier tubes produce an electrical pattern, which reflects the amount of radioactivity coming from the patient.

d) **False** The gamma rays absorbed by the crystal include some that were initially scattered in the patient, as well as others that lost energy via Compton interactions in the crystal before being absorbed. This means that the electrical energy produced by the camera varies. A pulse height analyser is used to count only energy pulses lying within a preset window (around 140 keV for ^{99m}Tc studies) in order to minimise the contribution of scatter or Compton interactions to the final image. The photopeak lies at the high-energy end of the pulse height spectrum and results from unscattered gamma rays.

e) **True** Spatial resolution is the ability of the camera to produce distinct images of two radioactive sources close together. Intrinsic resolution refers to the resolution of the camera, whilst system resolution is calculated after the gamma rays have also passed through the collimator and patient. System resolution is no better than one line pair per centimetre.

3 a) **True** The radionuclides used in PET scanning emit positrons that collide with nearby electrons and are annihilated, resulting in the release of two high energy (511 keV) photons that travel in opposite directions. These photons can be detected by opposing pairs of bismuth germinate detectors that form a ring around the patient. Any photon pulses that do not coincide in time are rejected. By having multiple pairs of detectors and by attaching the radionuclide to a known metabolic substrate, it is possible to construct a cross-sectional image of the metabolic activity within the patient.

  b) **True** Positron-emitting radionuclides are nearly all cyclotron-produced and, as most have a short half-life (^{18}FDG = 110 minutes), an on-site cyclotron is required.

  c) **True** PET uses electronic collimation instead of the lead collimators (which markedly reduce the number of photons reaching the detector) used in SPECT. Therefore, it has better resolution (approximately 2–5 mm) than SPECT (about 4–7 mm). PET spatial resolution is the same at all depths, unlike SPECT, which worsens with depth.

  d) **False** ^{18}FDG competes with glucose for cell entry. Once inside the cell, it behaves in a similar fashion to unlabelled glucose, but only takes part in the first step of the Kreb's cycle. It is, therefore, a good marker of glycolytic metabolic activity, which is elevated in many tumours, including lymphoma, which leads most neoplasms to appear as 'hot spots' on PET imaging.

  e) **True** As patients with diabetes usually have high circulating blood levels of glucose (unlabelled) and low insulin levels, there is decreased ^{18}FDG cell entry, resulting in less avid tissue uptake of radionuclide.

4 a) **True** ^{99m}Tc MDP is the most commonly used agent in bone scintigraphy. Unlike older agents, it is able to resist *in vivo* hydrolysis by alkaline phosphatase. Bone uptake depends on two factors: osteoblastic activity and blood flow.

  b) **True** Hence, the bladder receives a high radiation dose, which is reduced by good hydration and frequent voiding (this also prevents obscuration of pelvic lesions).

  c) **False** Static images are usually obtained after 2–4 hours, but can take longer in cases of renal insufficiency. In a four-phase study, images are acquired of flow (first 60 seconds), blood pool (1–5 minutes), static (2–4 hours) and delayed stages (24 hours).

  d) **False** Salivary gland uptake occurs secondary to free pertechnetate; uptake of which is also seen in the thyroid and stomach. Sites of increased MDP uptake in normal scans include: acromioclavicular, sacroiliac and sternoclavicular joints, costochondral junction(s), deltoid tuberosity (in 7% of scans), scapular tip, lower cervical spine, growth plates, muscle and tendon insertions (e.g. in line along the posterior ribs due to erector spinae muscles) and at sites of degenerative change. Patchy skull uptake can be normal. Strikingly 'hot' or asymmetrical sites are abnormal.

  e) **True** ^{99m}Tc MDP uptake also occurs in various extra-osseous locations: tissue infarction (myocardial, cerebral and splenic), cardiac insults (surgery, unstable angina and cardiomyopathies), soft-tissue calcification (myositis ossificans and nephrocalcinosis), effusions (ascitic, pleural and pericardial: due to malignancy, uraemia or infection), abscesses, inflammatory breast carcinoma, liver necrosis/metastases, pneumonia and amyloid deposits.

5 a) **False** Acute fractures are not normally 'hot' until after the first 24–48 hours (up to 72 hours in the elderly). In adults, bone uptake returns to normal in 1 year (rib fractures) to 3 years (elderly and long-bone fractures).

b) **False** Most bone islands do not take up MDP, but some (about 30%), especially if large, have a very slightly increased uptake. Other benign bone lesions that behave similarly include osteopoikilosis, osteopathia striata, fibrous cortical defect/nonossifying fibroma and haemangiomata.

c) **True** Numerous benign bone lesions can be 'hot' on a bone scan, including fibrous dysplasia, Paget's disease, brown tumours, aneurysmal bone cyst, Langerhans' cell histiocytosis, chondroblastoma, melorheostosis, osteoid osteoma, enchondroma and osteochondroma.

d) **True** Initially (in the first year), in more than 60% of cases of reflex sympathetic dystrophy, both blood pool and delayed images are 'hot'. Later, both of these images may become 'cold' on bone scans.

e) **False** However, with modern gamma cameras it is often possible to detect subtle areas of increased or decreased uptake in multiple myeloma.

6 All true A 'superscan' describes a bone scan in which there is a diffuse and symmetrical increase in bony uptake. There is usually almost total absence of renal or soft-tissue activity and bony uptake may be seen on the early blood pool images and in the sternum (the 'bow-tie' sign) and costochondral ('rosary beading') junctions. Causes of a superscan include:
- widespread bony metastases – primary sites include the prostate (most common), breast, lung, bladder, lymphoma and colon
- hyperparathyroidism
- osteomalacia (one may also see areas of more focal uptake in Looser's zones)
- renal osteodystrophy
- hyperthyroidism
- Paget's disease (usually a combination of 'hot' and 'cold' lesions)
- fibrous dysplasia
- mastocytosis
- myelofibrosis
- Waldenstrom's macroglobulinaemia
- aplastic anaemia/leukaemia

Uptake in a superscan in the calvarium and long bones makes a metabolic cause more likely than metastases, as the latter tends to spare these areas. In addition, unlike the diffuse uptake in metabolic disease, metastatic superscans tend to be slightly irregular.

7 a) **True**   This is known as the 'flare' phenomenon and is seen in 20%–60% of patients, typically 2–4 months after commencing chemotherapy. It reflects increased local blood flow and new bone formation secondary to healing. Presence or absence of a 'flare' has no prognostic significance. A follow-up scan in a further 3 months can help differentiate healing from progressive disease.

   b) **False**   The sclerotic component of an osteoid osteoma is usually 'hot' and the central nidus may be even hotter – the so-called 'double density' sign. This allows differentiation from osteomyelitis, in which the nidus is 'cold'.

   c) **True**   Although most malignant bony processes are 'hot', about 5% are 'cold', including multiple myeloma, purely lytic deposits, anaplastic tumours, infiltrating marrow lesions (histiocytosis and neuroblastoma) and some renal and thyroid cancer deposits (some of these conditions produce positive radiographs). Conversely, about 30%–50% of patients with a positive bone scan for metastases will have a normal radiograph.

   d) **False**   Radiotherapy causes an endarteritis, which decreases local blood flow and hence MDP uptake, leading to a 'cold' area with a well-defined border.

   e) **True**   Of the remaining nonmalignant lesions, 25% are due to trauma and 10% to infection. Location provides helpful information, as a peripheral lesion is less likely to be malignant; 80% of bony metastases are seen in the axial skeleton (35% in the ribs, 25% in the spine and 20% in the pelvis), 15% occur in the long bones and 5% in the skull.

8 a) **False**   Increased uptake over the greater and lesser trochanters is frequently seen in normal studies. Bursitis is suggested by increased uptake beyond the confines of bone on all phases of bone scan. Inflammatory bursitis is just one cause of a painful hip after a joint replacement. Other causes include prosthetic loosening and infection, heterotopic bone formation, breakage of fixation wires and fracture/dislocation of prosthesis. As some of these conditions are easily identified radiographically, plain film should be performed first.

   b) **True**   Cemented THRs remain 'hot' for only 6–12 months after surgery, but noncemented prostheses may be 'hot' for 24 months or longer.

   c) **False**   Unlike hip replacements, knee prostheses may remain 'hot' indefinitely. Therefore, bone scans are more accurate at assessing THRs than total knee replacements.

   d) **False**   Typically, infection causes hypervascularity and bony inflammation. Thus, images are 'hot' on both blood pool and delayed phases. Conversely, in prosthetic loosening, increased uptake is only seen in the delayed phase. Loosening usually causes increased uptake around the prosthetic tip, whereas infection results in diffuse uptake, but a white cell scan may be needed to differentiate between the two.

   e) **False**   Minor ^{67}Ga bony uptake around a prosthesis is nonspecific and can be seen normally and with loosening. If the amount of uptake is much greater than on concurrent MDP bone scan, infection is likely.

9 a) **True**   More than 90% of the injected dose is removed by the reticuloendothelial system (mainly the liver and spleen, obscuring images of the lower thoracic spine and ribs) and the remaining 10% localises in bone marrow. Bone marrow scans have a limited clinical role, but can show extramedullary haemopoiesis, guide red marrow biopsies and help identify bony infarcts in sickle cell anaemia ('cold' spots).

b) **False**   As these scans demonstrate active red marrow, any process that replaces normal marrow will show as a photopenic defect. Focal defects are also seen in infarction, osteomyelitis, radiotherapy and Paget's disease.

c) **False**   In normal adults, it is usual to see activity extending as far as the proximal third of the femur and humerus. Extension beyond this is abnormal. In neonates, red marrow extends to the peripheries, but with age the marrow retracts and adopts the adult pattern. Therefore, the scan appearance is age dependent.

d) **True**   There is decreased central activity (due to marrow fibrosis), but peripheral marrow hyperplasia is seen in 50% of patients. Peripheral marrow extension is also seen in all forms of haemolytic anaemia, Hodgkin's disease and polycythaemia rubra vera.

e) **True**   However, with recovery, normal central activity may be seen with peripheral extension. Other causes of reduced central marrow activity include: chronic myeloid leukaemia, myelofibrosis, chronic renal failure, lymphoma, multiple myeloma, metastases and radiotherapy.

10 a) **True**   Smaller particles may pass through the pulmonary capillaries and reach the systemic circulation. MAA acts by occluding pulmonary capillaries. More than 90% of injected particles are trapped in the lung on first pass. MAA particles should be less than 150 μm to avoid clumping.

b) **False**   MAA can still be used, but the dose needs to be reduced. The dose is also reduced in neonates and paediatric patients, in cases of pulmonary hypertension, patients on mechanical ventilation and critically ill patients with severe chronic obstructive airway disease (COAD).

c) **False**   A ventilation scan has to be performed first, as the Compton scatter from the ^{99m}Tc perfusion agent overlies the photopeak of the lower energy ^{133}Xe (81 keV). Despite this, ^{133}Xe is commonly used and it provides useful washout images (physical half-life = 5.2 days).

d) **True**   As a result of a short half-life, it must be breathed directly from a ^{81}rubidium generator and washout images cannot be obtained, limiting its sensitivity in obstructive lung disease. However, high emitted energy (190 keV) allows ventilation studies to be performed after a perfusion study.

e) **True**   Delivery is not as good as with gases and a large proportion of aerosolised particles deposit in the large central airways or are swallowed. Images may show focal 'hot' spots in the pharynx, tracheobronchial tree and stomach.

11 a) **True** This reflects greater perfusion to dependent parts of the lung in the supine patient. ^{99m}Tc MAA is injected supine to eliminate an apical-to-basal activity gradient.

 b) **False** The converse is true.

 c) **True** The stripe sign refers to an area of hypoperfusion with a zone of preserved peripheral perfusion. As pulmonary emboli are pleurally based, the presence of the stripe sign makes a pulmonary embolus unlikely. The defect is more likely to be due to COAD.

 d) **True** This was one of the criteria used in the Prospective Investigation of Pulmonary Embolism Diagnosis (PIOPED) study. In that study, scans were categorised as being normal or having a low, indeterminate or high probability for pulmonary emboli. The angiographic incidence of pulmonary emboli in each PIOPED category was 4%, 16%, 33% and 88%, respectively.

 e) **False** Pulmonary emboli typically appear as mismatched defects. A reversed mismatch (normal perfusion and abnormal ventilation) is more typical of atelectasis, pleural effusion, COAD or pneumonia. Other causes of a matched defect include old pulmonary emboli, other emboli, tuberculosis, vasculitis, radiotherapy, pulmonary hypertension and bronchogenic cancer.

12 All true This pattern is seen in approximately 2% of V/Q scans. The causes include the following.
Arterial disease
 • Massive pulmonary embolism
 • Swyer–James (Macleod's) syndrome (gives a matched defect)
 • Congenital pulmonary artery hypoplasia/stenosis
 • Shunt procedures to the pulmonary artery (e.g. Blalock–Taussig shunt)
 • Secondary to fibrosing mediastinitis (e.g. histoplasmosis, tuberculosis)
Airway disease (usually a small amount of perfusion can be identified)
 • Foreign-body obstruction
 • Bronchial carcinoma/adenoma
 • Bullous emphysema
 • Mucous plug
Pleural disease
 • Large pleural effusion
 • Pneumothorax
Absent lung
 • Pneumonectomy
 • Pulmonary agenesis
Congenital heart disease

13 a) **True** Cellular uptake is analogous to potassium uptake, but ^{201}Tl is less readily released from cells. Approximately 3%–4% of the total dose is extracted by the heart at rest, but uptake can be increased to 10% with pharmacological stress. The distribution of activity reflects regional cardiac blood flow and the integrity of the Na$^+$/K$^+$ ATPase pump. Peak cardiac activity occurs 5–15 minutes after injection.

b) **True** The long physical and biological half-life (approximately 10 days) limits the dose of ^{201}Tl (80 keV) that can be administered.

c) **True** The combination of a shorter half-life, permitting a higher injected dose, and higher energy (140 keV) photons from ^{99m}Tc leads to a higher photon flux in obese patients. ^{99m}Tc sestamibi has a high first-pass extraction, a distribution proportional to blood flow and few metabolic side-effects.

d) **True** This results in a need for separate stress and rest injections, unlike with ^{201}Tl chloride, which undergoes redistribution, permitting combined stress and rest imaging on the same day.

e) **True** This fact, coupled with the very rapid myocardial clearance of ^{99m}Tc teboroxime, necessitates imaging immediately (1–2 minutes) after injection and, thus, limits its versatility. It also undergoes some hepatobiliary excretion, which may interfere with inferior-wall evaluation.

14 a) **True** This is to limit splanchnic blood flow, as splanchnic uptake can be seen after a recent meal, inadequate exercise and after studies using dipyridamole or 2-methoxyisobutylisonitrile (MIBI). If cardiac stress is induced using dipyridamole, caffeine is restricted for 24 hours, as this can negate dipyridamole's vasodilator effect.

b) **False** The target heart rate is 85% of the predicted maximum heart rate, which is calculated as 220 minus the patient's age in years. The endpoints on a treadmill test are attaining target heart rate, completing the exercise protocol (e.g. modified Bruce), onset of fatigue or dyspnoea preventing continuation of the test, or the development of cardiovascular signs or symptoms (such as severe angina, hypotension, arrhythmias and ischaemia on electrocardiogram [ECG]).

c) **True** One disadvantage of using exercise to induce cardiac stress is that about 35% of patients fail to reach their target heart rate, with a consequent drop in test sensitivity for ischaemia. Despite this, exercise is generally preferred over pharmacological stress testing, as only exercise leads to a significant increase in cardiac workload. Ischaemia is seldom seen after pharmacological stress.

d) **True** If the ratio is more than 0.5, left ventricular dysfunction should be suspected.

e) **False** Adenosine can cause bronchospasm and, thus, is contraindicated in patients with asthma or those who use inhalers. Other recognised side-effects include flushing, heart block and nausea. These side-effects often dissipate rapidly after stopping adenosine infusion, as the half-life is only 15 seconds. Bronchospasm can also be seen after use of dipyridamole, but can be reversed by giving intravenous aminophylline. The agent of choice in patients with asthma is dobutamine.

15 All true There are three basic patterns on a ^{201}Tl stress test.
- Reversible perfusion defect is a perfusion defect on the stress images that partially or totally fills-in on the rest images. The most common cause is ischaemia, but it is also rarely seen in Chagas' disease, sarcoidosis and hypertrophic cardiomyopathy.
- Irreversible perfusion defect is a perfusion defect seen on stress images that persists on rest images. It is often seen with old myocardial infarctions, cardiomyopathies, idiopathic subaortic stenosis and infiltrative and metastatic lesions.
- A rapid washout pattern on stress view appears normal, but a defect is seen on redistribution images. It is nonspecific, but may occur in coronary artery disease, cardiomyopathy or in normal individuals.

Hibernating myocardium is myocardium that shows absent wall motion and reduced or absent blood flow, but which, following a revascularisation procedure, may regain function. On ^{201}Tl images, it may resemble an area of infarction, but it has been shown that images obtained after a second ^{201}Tl injection or after 24 hours may show some uptake, thereby differentiating the hibernating from the infarcted myocardium.

16 a) False Cardiac PET studies usually rely on pharmacological stress testing, as exercise is difficult to perform whilst in the scanner.

b) True [82]Rubidium is a marker of myocardial blood flow that is similar to Tl. It can be produced from a [82]strontium/[82]rubidium generator, meaning an on-site generator is not necessary. The physical half-life is only 76 seconds, allowing repeat blood-flow measurements within short time intervals. [13]Nitrogen (half-life = 10 minutes) is also a marker of myocardial blood flow, but is produced in a cyclotron.

c) False In myocardial ischaemia, there is an increase in glycolysis (and, therefore, uptake of glucose) with a decrease in the usual oxidation of fatty acids. Hence, [18]FDG imaging provides information about myocardial metabolism.

d) False PET is probably the noninvasive test of choice for identifying hibernating myocardium (dysfunctional myocardium that regains function after revascularisation). On PET, it is characterised by decreased perfusion, but enhanced [18]FDG metabolism (a mismatched defect). PET is more sensitive than ^{201}Tl in detecting hibernating myocardium.

e) True Areas with decreased perfusion and metabolism (a matched defect) are likely to reflect previous infarction or fibrosis. They indicate nonviable myocardium and only 10%–20% will regain function after revascularisation.

17 a) **False** There are two kinds of scintigraphic ventricular function test: 'first-pass' and 'gated red blood pool' studies. ^{99m}Tc DTPA is the radiotracer used in first-pass studies, whilst ^{99m}Tc-labelled red cells are used in gated blood pool studies. ^{99m}Tc DTPA cannot be used for gated studies because its blood clearance by glomerular filtration is too rapid to allow prolonged imaging.

b) **True** In this kind of shunt, refilling of the right ventricle and lungs is noted. Right-to-left shunts are also easily detected. First-pass studies allow determination of transit time and right ventricular ejection fraction; the latter is often difficult to detect with gated blood pool studies because of overlap of activity in the right atrium and pulmonary artery. These studies involve imaging the heart, lungs and great vessels immediately after the injection of radiotracer. The image acquisition ends before the agent recirculates.

c) **True** In blood pool studies, the image acquisition is gated to the R-wave of the cardiac cycle. This test provides optimal assessment of segmental wall motion and is the test of choice for LVEF determination; it is more accurate than echocardiography or contrast ventriculography. Ventricular wall motion is graded segmentally and segments should contract simultaneously. Typically, the anterior, posterior and lateral walls move to a greater extent than the septum or inferior wall.

d) **True** Normal variability is 5%. Cardiotoxicity should be suspected if the ejection fraction falls by more than 10% on sequential scans on patients receiving chemotherapy and treatment should be stopped. The absolute value of ejection fraction is also important, as some treatments (such as adriamycin) are stopped if the ejection fraction falls below 45%.

e) **False** Normally, LVEF increases by at least 5% with exercise, but patients with coronary artery disease or those aged over 60 years may show a fall or no increase.

18 a) **False** It is mostly cleared by tubular secretion. It undergoes minimal (10%) glomerular filtration and this makes it an effective renal plasma flow agent. It is not retained in the renal parenchyma.

b) **True** This is because it is not reliant on glomerular filtration. Thus, in the setting of renal impairment, there is still high renal extraction and a good tissue-to-background ratio. In renal insufficiency, there may be some hepato-biliary excretion of MAG$_3$ with visualisation of the liver, biliary tree and small bowel.

c) **True** It is entirely cleared by glomerular filtration, making it a useful agent for measuring the glomerular filtration rate (GFR); as it is 5%–10% protein bound, the calculated GFR is lower than with inulin. It undergoes no tubular secretion. Immediate images provide information about renal perfusion, whilst delayed images provide information about GFR and the collecting system. It is less expensive than MAG$_3$.

d) **False** DMSA may overestimate renal function, as excreted tracer in the obstructed collecting system will contribute to renal activity. MAG$_3$ is preferred.

e) **True** This is why ^{99m}Tc DMSA provides such good images of the renal cortex, but offers little information about renal function or excretion. Other disadvantages include a high radiation dose and limited availability. It is used in the assessment of renal scarring in children (SPECT increases sensitivity) and differentiating renal pseudotumour (made up of functioning renal tissue) from a mass lesion.

19 a) **True**   Perfusion (flow) images are rapid sequential images acquired over the first minute. The aorta is normally seen first. Images are acquired with the patient supine or prone, as the upright position can lead to anterior displacement of the upper pole, foreshortening the kidney. Renal perfusion and size should be symmetrical.

b) **True**   After a peak at 3–5 minutes, cortical activity decreases with time.

c) **True**   In renal impairment, splenic or liver activity may be greater than renal activity.

d) **False**   Split renal function is determined with a region of interest (ROI) cursor over each kidney, with adjustments made for background activity. Measurements are made after 2–3 minutes, before the collecting systems start to fill. The collecting system and ureters should begin to fill after 4–5 minutes.

e) **False**   Persistent visualisation of a ureter is abnormal, but transient visualisation, especially on a MAG$_3$ study, is normal.

20 a) **False**   In order to maintain a positive glomerular filtration pressure in the setting of renal artery stenosis, there is constriction of the efferent arteriole, a process mediated via the renin–angiotensin pathway. Following the use of ACE inhibitors, this pathway is blocked and the efferent arteriole dilates, the filtration pressure falls and the amount of isotope filtered or taken up by that kidney is reduced. Acute renal failure can be induced by this test in the presence of a single kidney with severe renal artery stenoses, or in bilateral severe RAS.

b) **True**   In addition, ACE inhibitors should be stopped for at least 2 days before the test and the patient should be well hydrated to minimise the hypotensive effect of the ACE inhibitor and limit the radiation dose to the bladder.

c) **False**   Differential diagnoses for this appearance include RSA, renal vein thrombosis, unilateral acute tubular necrosis and glomerulonephritis, perirenal abscess, or haematoma and an obstructive uropathy.

d) **False**   Bilateral disease, which is seen in 30% of cases of renovascular hypertension, may lead to a false negative study, as the split renal uptake of isotope will not change if both renal arteries are involved. However, one artery is usually more severely affected, allowing post-ACE inhibitor asymmetry to be detected.

e) **False**   A positive MAG$_3$ RAS renogram typically demonstrates a continually rising activity curve. A rise in cortical activity of more than 10% on 20-minute post-MAG$_3$ images is consistent with a significant stenosis.

21 a) True There are two techniques for radionuclide cystography: direct and indirect. Direct cystography involves instillation of ^{99m}Tc pertechnetate directly into the bladder via a urethral catheter, whilst indirect cystography is performed following intravenous administration of ^{99m}Tc DTPA. The direct technique is more sensitive for reflux during the bladder-filling phase.

b) False In virtually all patients with vesico-ureteric reflux, some degree of reflux will be seen during micturition. In about 80% of cases, vesico-ureteric reflux also occurs during the filling phase.

c) False Most patients will demonstrate a bladder volume below that at which reflux occurs (the threshold volume). Typically, on serial studies this volume increases as the ureteric orifice matures.

d) True The most commonly used fluoroscopic grading system (a 1–5 scale) requires subtle assessment of the fornices and collecting system that is not possible on scintigraphy. However, isotope studies can accurately quantify the amount of reflux and, therefore, provide prognostic information. Reflux just into the distal ureter is likely to resolve spontaneously, whereas reflux in the presence of a tortuous dilated ureter will require surgery.

e) True If renal scarring has not occurred by this age, the reflux is not significant.

22 a) True Acute tubular necrosis is the most common form of acute, reversible renal failure in transplant patients. It is usually seen in the first 24 hours and is rare after the first month. Imaging shows smooth, enlarged kidneys with normal or only slightly diminished MAG$_3$ perfusion, but much diminished excretion. Cyclosporin toxicity can have a similar appearance, but typically occurs after the first month.

b) True In acute rejection, excretion is always reduced, but perfusion may initially be normal. Serial studies may be required to differentiate this from acute tubular necrosis. Hyperacute rejection, which is rare and results from preformed antibodies from an earlier failed transplant, may demonstrate absent perfusion and excretion, necessitating immediate surgery.

c) True Other vascular complications include: renal vein thrombosis (which usually occurs in the first 3 days after transplant), RSA (the findings of which are similar to those in a native kidney), renal infarction and pseudoaneurysm formation.

d) False Urinomas usually develop during the first month posttransplant and may be 'cold' on scintigraphy for several reasons. Firstly, the leak may not be active at the time of study. Secondly, most leaks occur near the vesico-ureteric junction and may be obscured by the bladder; thus, postmicturition views are essential. Finally, urinomas may lead to hydronephrosis and renal impairment, reducing isotope excretion and, hence, the chance of visualising a urinoma.

e) False Both appear initially as extrarenal photopenic areas, but on delayed images the urinoma may, unlike a haematoma, show accumulation of activity. A haematoma may not be distinguishable from a lymphocoele.

23 a) **False** Liquids can exit the stomach purely by gravity, whereas solids have to first be reduced in size by stomach peristalsis before relying on antral contractions to enter the small bowel. This test, although not frequently performed, can provide useful information about possible gastroparesis (e.g. in patients with diabetes mellitus) or dumping syndrome. The usual isotope is ^{99m}Tc sulphur colloid.

b) **False** The stomach handles liquids and solids differently. Liquids empty faster and show a monophasic exponential clearance. Solids empty after an initial delay, but the emptying is nearly linear. Slower emptying occurs with large meals, high calorie meals and in premenopausal females (due to a progesterone effect).

c) **True** The emptying half-time for solids is usually 1–2 hours.

d) **False** Typically, emptying is delayed in anorexia nervosa. It is also delayed in mechanical gastric outlet obstruction, diabetes mellitus, scleroderma, dermatomyositis, hypokalaemia, uraemia, hypothyroidism, myotonia dystrophica, postsurgery (e.g. vagotomy without adequate drainage procedure), amyloidosis and secondary to drugs (e.g. beta-blockers, anticholinergic agents, opiates) or pain.

e) **True** Other causes of rapid emptying include postsurgery (e.g. antrectomy, gastrectomy and vagotomy when performed with adequate drainage procedure), coeliac disease, Zollinger–Ellison syndrome and duodenal ulcer disease.

24 a) **True** Patients who are asymptomatic throughout childhood are less likely to have a diverticulum containing ectopic gastric mucosa, which is necessary for detection by pertechnetate scintigraphy. Overall, 30%–50% of diverticula contain ectopic gastric mucosa. Of these, 60% contain ectopic gastric mucosa if the patient is symptomatic (symptoms usually occur before the age of 2 years) and 90% if they are bleeding. Ectopic gastric mucosa is present in only 5%–20% of Meckel's diverticula, but this percentage rises to 60% if the patient is symptomatic and 90% if they are bleeding.

b) **False** Activity in the diverticulum will first appear at the same time as pertechnetate accumulates in the normal gastric mucosa (5–20 minutes postinjection).

c) **False** Glucagon is often administered because it decreases peristalsis and so prevents downstream washout of pertechnetate. It also decreases pertechnetate uptake, which is undesirable, but it can be coadministered with pentagastrin, which increases pertechnetate uptake. Other pharmacological agents that can be used include: pentagrastin, which enhances gastric mucosal uptake of pertechnetate, and cimetidine and ranitidine, both of which inhibit intraluminal secretion and potential translocation of pertechnetate into the small bowel.

d) **False** Typically, uptake is focal and not tubular. Even though the diverticulum is tubular, the ectopic gastric mucosa normally only affects a small area of tissue. Tubular activity is more typical of the bowel.

e) **True** Any cause of ectopic gastric mucosa (e.g. enteric duplication, gastrogenic cyst) can simulate a Meckel's diverticulum. Other causes of a false positive scan include: normal activity in the bowel, bladder or kidneys; local inflammation, such as appendicitis and intussusception; hypervascularity of a tumour, aneurysm or arteriovenous malformation; calyceal diverticulum and urinary tract obstruction. Causes of false negative scans include: small size; absent/necrosed gastric mucosa; rapid downstream washout of tracer; obscuration by overlying structures.

25 a) **True** Angiography can detect bleeding rates of greater than 0.5 ml/min, while isotope studies may detect rates as low as 0.05–0.1 ml/min.

b) **True** Therefore, studies using ^{99m}Tc-labelled red cells are more sensitive for intermittent bleeding than those using ^{99m}Tc sulphur colloid or angiography. In addition to the rate of bleeding and whether bleeding is intermittent, test sensitivities also depend on the site of bleeding and the isotope agent used (see below).

c) **False** On sulphur colloid studies, in which label is taken up by the reticuloendothelial system, there is usually high activity in the liver and spleen. This obscures most of the proximal small bowel, making it difficult to detect gastric or duodenal bleeding. The hepatic and splenic flexures of the large bowel are also obscured.

d) **False** GI bleeding typically changes location with time as the extravasated blood moves along the bowel and continued bleeding leads to an increase in activity. Nonmoving bowel activity may indicate a colitis, as uptake is seen in colitis from inflammatory bowel disease, ischaemia and radiotherapy, or may indicate faulty labelling, leading to free pertechnetate being excreted into the bowel.

e) **True** This syndrome is characterised by multisystem telangectasias and arteriovenous malformations in the bowel and haemangiomas in the liver. Any abnormal vascular structure (e.g. arteriovenous malformations, varices, aneurysms, haemangiomas) may take up isotope and mimic GI bleeding thereby limiting the test specificity.

26 a) **True** These agents are cleared from plasma by hepatocytes with a blood half-life of only 10–20 minutes and are excreted in a similar fashion to bile. The degree of urinary excretion may be higher in patients with hepatic or biliary dysfunction.

b) **True** On a normal study, the liver should be visualised on early images and the gallbladder and duodenum should be seen by 1 hour postinjection. If the gallbladder is not seen, delayed images (for up to 24 hours) may help differentiate between acute (the gallbladder almost never fills) and chronic cholecystitis (delayed filling is usual).

c) **True** If the gallbladder is seen after the duodenum, it may indicate chronic cholecystitis. Another sign suggesting chronic cholecystitis is prolonged biliary-to-bowel transit time. If only the bowel is not seen, consider choledocholithiasis or ampullary stenosis.

d) **False** Two pharmacological manoeuvres can be used to aid in visualising the gallbladder if it is not seen on the initial images. Firstly, cholecystokinin (CCK) administration causes gallbladder contraction, which may allow it to re-fill if it is initially distended from prolonged fasting; some centres give CCK routinely to all patients fasted for longer than 24 hours. Secondly, morphine contracts the sphincter of Oddi and forces excreted IDA into the gallbladder, if the cystic duct is patent.

e) **False** The width of the common bile duct on images reflects the amount of radioactivity in the duct from excreted ^{99m}Tc IDA, rather than its actual size. Estimates of duct patency are made from distribution of activity rather than duct size.

27 a) **True** Other causes of failure to visualise the gallbladder at 4 hours include: acute and chronic cholecystitis; prolonged fasting; a recent meal, which causes the gallbladder to contract; total parenteral nutrition; severe intercurrent disease (including pancreatitis and hepatitis); and cystic duct cholangiocarcinoma. Delayed 24-hour images may be helpful.

b) **False** This refers to a rim of increased activity in the liver parenchyma adjacent to the gallbladder in cholecystitis. Possible causes include a local increase in liver blood flow and delayed drainage of excreted IDA secondary to oedema.

c) **True** Classically, acute cholecystitis is characterised by failure to visualise the gallbladder on all phases of the study due to complete blockage of the cystic duct. However, in about 4% of cases of acute cholecystitis, there is incomplete cystic duct obstruction and the gallbladder is seen on delayed images. In these circumstances, the appearance is indistinguishable from chronic cholecystitis.

d) **True** Duodenal diverticula can cause false negative studies as the diverticulum can be confused with the gallbladder. An accessory cystic duct is another cause of a false negative study, as it may allow gallbladder filling, even if the other duct is blocked.

e) **False** They both cause delayed gallbladder visualisation. The clinical setting may provide clues, as acalculous cholecystitis is more common in trauma, burns and on intensive care units.

28 a) **False** Some forms of this rare condition can be treated with a portoenterostomy (Kasai) procedure. This has a 90% success rate in the first 2 months of life, 50% in the third month and less than 20% after 3 months. Thus, a HIDA scan is best performed early, before irreversible liver damage occurs. If the test is delayed, liver function is so impaired secondary to biliary cirrhosis that it is often difficult to distinguish between neonatal hepatitis and biliary atresia.

b) **False** Phenobarbitone is frequently administered for 5 days preceding a HIDA test in order to induce liver enzymes (and to improve agent conjugation and excretion), as liver function is often impaired in these patients.

c) **True** If the liver is not seen on early images and/or there is delayed clearance from blood pool and some bowel activity after 24 hours, neonatal hepatitis should be suspected. If there is good liver activity on early images, but no bowel activity on 24-hour images with or without increased renal excretion, biliary atresia should be considered.

d) **True** Choledochal cysts communicate with the biliary tree and are, therefore, seen on HIDA scans, unlike pancreatic cysts, which cannot be detected unless their size causes some degree of biliary obstruction.

e) **True** There is frequently abdominal free fluid after biliary surgery, which limits the specificity of ultrasound, but it will only show on a HIDA scan if it contains bile.

29 a) True ^{123}I is the isotope of choice for several reasons. Firstly, it is not only trapped by the thyroid, but also undergoes organification and, therefore, the distribution of ^{123}I activity reflects thyroid function. Secondly, compared with ^{131}I and ^{99m}Tc pertechnetate, it has a better target-to-background ratio and a lower whole-body dose, although the dose to the thyroid is higher than with pertechnetate. It is also trapped in the stomach and salivary glands.

b) False ^{123}I is usually administered orally (4–8 MBq of sodium iodide tablets) as it is readily absorbed from the GI tract. Imaging is performed 24 hours later.

c) True ^{99m}Tc pertechnetate is rapidly trapped by the thyroid, but is not organified, and so it does not provide the same functional information as ^{123}I. It is quickly released, with virtually no isotope left in the gland at 24 hours. It also accumulates in the salivary glands, stomach and choroid plexus. It is used in place of ^{123}I if imaging is to be performed within 1 hour, if the patient is taking propylthiouracil, which blocks organification, or if the patient is not able to ingest iodine orally.

d) True ^{131}I emits β rays, which are responsible for 90% of the radiation, and γ rays and is now only used for the detection and ablation of thyroid metastases and therapeutically in Grave's disease. The long half-life requires long patient isolation. Its use may be complicated by sialoadenitis, nausea and vomiting, leukaemia, breast and bladder cancer (both rare), bone marrow depression or sterility if there are pelvic thyroid carcinoma metastases.

e) False ^{99m}Tc and ^{123}I are as capable at demonstrating retrosternal thyroid tissue and have none of the inherent disadvantages of ^{131}I. However, ^{123}I is superior to ^{99m}Tc pertechnetate for confirming the presence of lingual thyroid tissue, as more marked ^{99m}Tc pertechnetate salivary gland uptake obscures images.

30 a) False Nodules can be defined as 'hot', 'warm' or 'cold' depending on their activity relative to normal thyroid. The vast majority of 'hot' nodules represent hyperfunctioning adenomas, whereas 10% of 'warm' nodules are malignant. Ideally, nodules should be described as 'indeterminate', rather than 'warm', to avoid confusion with 'hot' nodules.

b) True About 90% of palpable nodules are 'cold' and of these up to 90% are benign. A 'cold' nodule may represent an adenoma/colloid cyst (85%), carcinoma (10%), focal thyroiditis, lymph node, haemorrhage, abscess or parathyroid adenoma. The incidence of malignancy in a solitary thyroid nodule rises to 30%–50% if there is a previous history of childhood head and neck irradiation. Other factors that increase the risk of malignancy within a nodule include: age under 20 or over 60 years, male sex, family history of thyroid carcinoma, dysphagia, rapid growth, single nodule and lymphadenopathy.

c) False Only 10% are palpable, even when their position is known from imaging.

d) True The risk of underlying carcinoma in a dominant nodule is low (less than 5%), but the risk of malignancy anywhere in a multinodular gland is as high as 13% in some series.

e) True A discordant nodule is nonfunctioning (i.e. 'cold' on ^{123}I) and usually reflects a thyroid adenoma with a disrupted organification pathway.

31 a) **False**   The thyroid uptake test determines how much of an orally ingested dose of ^{123}I has accumulated within the thyroid gland at 24 hours. It is, therefore, a measure of iodine trapping and organification. Normal values are 10%–30% of the oral dose. Increased values are seen in: thyrotoxicosis (e.g. Grave's disease), iodine deficiency, hypoalbuminaemia and lithium use. Decreased uptake is seen with hypothyroidism and secondary to the use of various drugs, such as thyroid hormone replacement therapy, thyroid-blocking therapy and glucocorticoids.

    b) **True**   Thyroiditis can cause increased or decreased uptake.

    c) **False**   Low tracer uptake occurs in a number of hyperthyroid states, including amiodarone-induced thyrotoxicosis, subacute or postpartum thyroiditis, recent heavy iodine load (e.g. recent contrast media), excessive thyroxine administration or ectopic hyperfunctioning tissue. This condition is worth recognising, as hyperthyroidism will not respond to radioiodine treatment.

    d) **False**   This is known as the 'owl's eye sign'; the 'cold' area almost always represents an area of cystic degeneration within a solitary functioning nodule. The reversed pattern, with peripheral photopenia and a central 'hot' spot, also suggests benignity and is known as the 'fish eye sign', which usually reflects peripheral cystic change in a functioning adenoma.

    e) **True**   Some studies have suggested that thyroglobulin levels are as sensitive as ^{131}I at detecting residual/recurrent malignant thyroid tissue.

32 a) **False**   [201]Tl localises to both normal thyroid tissue and enlarged parathyroid glands, whereas ^{99m}Tc pertechnetate is taken up by the thyroid gland only. By performing these two tests together and electronically subtracting the images, it is possible to obtain images of the parathyroid glands.

    b) **True**   This is because ^{201}Tl may also accumulate in benign thyroid adenomas, lymph nodes, thyroid carcinomas and rarely in sarcoidosis and lymphoma. [201]Tl scans may be uninterpretable in the presence of a multinodular goitre.

    c) **True**   The exact cause of this is unclear, but it may be because adenomas tend to be larger than hyperplastic glands. The sensitivity for detecting adenomas is 70%–90%, but this is very dependent on the lesion size and location. Adenomas are rarely identified if they are smaller than 0.5 g and sensitivity is higher for ectopic tissue.

    d) **True**   [99m]Tc sestamibi is taken up by both thyroid and parathyroid tissue, but it quickly washes out of thyroid tissue. On delayed images, parathyroid adenomas persist as focal 'hot' spots.

    e) **True**   Due to the more favourable physical characteristics of ^{99m}Tc sestamibi (principal γ emission of 140 keV and half-life = 6 hours) compared with [201]Tl (principal γ emission of 80, 135 and 167 keV and half-life = 73 hours), as well as the simple protocol (early and delayed imaging) and no need for prolonged patient immobilisation due to a reduced risk of movement artefact, many centres have replaced ^{201}Tl/^{99m}Tc subtraction scans with sestamibi scanning for imaging the parathyroid glands.

33 a) **False** This lipophilic agent freely passes through the blood–brain barrier and is trapped in neurones for several hours after intravenous administration, secondary to an intracellular reaction with glutathione, which converts it to a nonlipophilic moiety. Normal brain activity is maximal 1 minute postinjection. Activity plateaus after 2 minutes and then remains constant for about 8 hours.

   b) **False** The reverse is true. Uptake is also seen in the liver and renal tract, as well as in the lungs of smokers and occasionally in lung cancer.

   c) **True** Reduced basal ganglia flow is also seen in Fahr's and Wilson's diseases. Conversely, in Parkinson's disease, there is increased basal ganglia activity.

   d) **True** Typically, in Alzheimer's disease, there are bilateral perfusion defects in the parietal lobes, as well as in the temporal, occipital and frontal lobes. This process spares the visual and sensorimotor cortex, subcortical regions and cerebellum, which results in a reduction of the cortical/cerebellar uptake ratio from a normal of 1 to less than 0.8. The main differential diagnosis is multi-infarct dementia, which shows asymmetrical perfusion defects. ^{99m}Tc HMPAO can also be used for brain-death studies: it is positive for brain death if it shows no flow or uptake in the brain.

   e) **True** During a seizure, there is increased uptake at the site of the seizure focus. Seizure studies are conducted in a dark and quiet room with the patient still. Due to the short *in vivo* stability of HMPAO (about 30 minutes), seizures often have to be induced postinjection.

34 a) **False** The converse is true. ^{67}Ga is bound to iron transport proteins, such as transferrin, ferritin and lactoferrin, which bind at sites of infection. This property, along with its uptake in neutrophils, helps ^{67}Ga to be taken up by a wide variety of inflammatory and neoplastic conditions. However, in patients with saturated iron-binding sites (e.g. haemochromatosis), there is increased renal excretion, resulting in decreased soft-tissue localisation.

   b) **True** This is because ^{67}Ga uptake into neutrophils is partly responsible for its ability to localise inflammation or a tumour (see above). Other common causes of a false negative scan include a small area of inflammation, the affected area not being imaged or uptake being obscured by overlying organs, such as the colon.

   c) **False** The principal sites of normal localisation of ^{67}Ga are in the liver, spleen, bone marrow and bone. Transient uptake is normally seen in the kidneys (for 24 hours), the colon (for more than 24 hours) and the following for 6–24 hours: the lacrimal and salivary glands, nasal mucosa, external genitalia, thymus and breast tissue (especially during pregnancy, with the oral contraceptive pill and during menarche). Infants demonstrate significant activity in the base of the skull and the eipiphyses, as do children.

   d) **False** Although initially renally excreted, with faint activity sometimes seen in the kidneys up to 48 hours postinjection, renal activity after 72 hours is always abnormal. After 24 hours, the colon becomes the major route of excretion, which limits the usefulness of ^{67}Ga in abdominal imaging.

   e) **True** The physical half-life is 78 hours and the blood half-life is 12 hours. Images are obtained 24–72 hours after intravenous administration. Photopeaks are seen at 93, 185 and 300 keV.

35 a) **False** Kaposi's sarcoma does not usually take up ^{67}Ga.

b) **True** A ^{67}Ga scan is abnormal in 85%–95% of cases. A normal ^{67}Ga scan and chest X-ray make *P. carinii* pneumonia very unlikely. There is often increased uptake at a time when physical signs, symptoms and radiographic changes are minimal. Other causes of gallium uptake and a normal chest X-ray include drug toxicity, (such as bleomycin and amiodarone), tumour infiltration and sarcoidosis.

c) **True** A ^{67}Ga scan is 95% sensitive for detecting mediastinal disease lymphoma. It is most accurate for the nodular sclerosing and least accurate for the lymphocyte- predominant subtypes of mediastinal lymphoma.

d) **True** Typically, in pneumonia there is a segmental or lobar pattern of uptake. Uptake is also seen in other infections, such as cytomegalovirus pneumonia, *Cryptococcus* infection, tuberculosis (uptake reflects disease activity) and toxoplasmosis.

e) **True** ^{67}Ga scans are 70% sensitive for active parenchymal disease and 95% sensitive for hilar adenopathy. ^{67}Ga uptake indicates a likely response to steroids. Other inflammatory conditions that take up ^{67}Ga include: idiopathic pulmonary fibrosis, pneumoconiosis, lymphangitis, and exudative radiation pneumonitis. The most common chest uses of ^{67}Ga are to assess sarcoidosis activity, the early detection of *P. carinii* pneumonia and in lymphoma staging, as it can differentiate between residual disease and inactive fibrosis. Its role in staging lung carcinoma is controversial; it will detect 90% of tumours and those missed are usually less than 2 cm. Sensitivities in this role have varied from 30% to 100%. It is possibly less sensitive for adenocarcinoma.

36 a) **True** These type of scans are performed to identify areas of inflammation or infection. The most common label in white cell imaging is ^{111}In oxine. The lipophilic oxine component allows ^{111}In to enter the white cell; the bond is then broken and ^{111}In binds intracellularly and oxine leaves the cell. Another white cell label is ^{99m}Tc HMPAO, which allows earlier imaging than ^{111}In oxine (1–4 hours versus 18–24 hours), but suffers from bowel excretion and the fact that the heart and blood pool activity may obscure underlying disease. Other compounds sometimes used in this kind of imaging include ^{67}Ga citrate, ^{111}In IgG and chemotactic peptides.

b) **True** This is because ^{67}Ga citrate is excreted via the colon and the activity in the faeces potentially obscures any abdominal pathology. In addition, the colon is usually seen at 24 hours on ^{99m}Tc HMPAO white cell studies. The GI tract or kidneys are not normally seen on a ^{111}In oxine-labelled white cell study.

c) **True** This is in contrast to a ^{67}Ga citrate scan, in which the liver is 'hotter' than the spleen. On a ^{111}In oxine study, the spleen receives the highest radiation dose.

d) **False** It is often normal on both ^{111}In oxine and ^{99m}Tc HMPAO studies to see the lungs on images acquired in the first 4 hours. The exact reason for this is unclear, but may reflect physiological white cell margination in the pulmonary circulation or possibly pulmonary repair of white cells damaged during labelling.

e) **False** Usually this is true, but in severe leucopenia, when there may not be enough cells to label, donor blood may be used.

37 a) **False** There are many other causes of a false positive study (i.e. no actual infection) including surgical scars that are at least 10 days old, intravenous injection sites, colostomies, accessory spleen, haematomas, active bleeding, myocardial infarcts, cerebrovascular accidents, necrotic bowel, myocarditis, pancreatitis, rejected renal transplants, sinusitis, tumours, fractures (for the first 2 weeks) and bowel activity secondary to swallowed purulent material from disease in the lungs, sinuses or mouth. An abscess (a true positive study) appears as a focal area of activity that is equal to or hotter than the liver and that becomes hotter on delayed images.

   b) **False** A chronic abscess may become walled off and so prevent or delay entry of labelled white cells, resulting in a false negative study; this is more of a problem with ^{99m}Tc HMPAO because images are acquired early. Other causes of a false negative study include agranulocytosis, immunosuppression, steroid use and acute spinal osteomyelitis (the exact reason for the latter is not clear).

   c) **False** Ulcerative colitis, Crohn's disease and infective colitis are all 'hot'. With white cells labelled with ^{99m}Tc HMPAO, bowel activity is seen in normal individuals on 24-hour images. Thus, images have to be acquired early (1–4 hours).

   d) **True** Other noninfective causes of lung activity include congestive heart failure, pulmonary emboli, adult respiratory distress syndrome and atelectasis. Lung activity is, therefore, less specific for infection, as up to one sixth of all studies will show activity in the lungs.

   e) **False** Although this would seem logical, studies have shown no significant effect of concurrent antibiotic usage on white cell study sensitivity.

38 All true MIBG labelled with radioactive iodine (^{123}I or ^{131}I) localises in neuroendocrine tissue. It can therefore be used to localise neuroendocrine tumours, such as paraganglioma (e.g. phaeochromocytoma) carcinoid (primary and metastatic), medullary thyroid carcinoma, neuroblastoma, and ganglioneuroma. Normal structures that may be 'hot' on MIBG scans include the myocardium, adrenal glands, liver, spleen, bladder, salivary glands, thyroid, nasopharynx and colon. Faint visualisation of the adrenal medulla is seen in 16% of studies (more commonly with ^{123}I), but intense adrenal uptake is always abnormal. Bilateral adrenal uptake suggests hyperplasia, but unilateral uptake suggests a neuroendocrine tumour. Thyroid uptake of free iodine is blocked by pretest administration of potassium iodide. Images are acquired 4 and 24 hours after ^{123}I and 1–3 days after ^{131}I administration.

39 All true   Octreotide is a synthetic cyclic octapeptide with similar pharmacological properties to somatostatin and which can be labelled either with ^{123}I or [111]In. It has a half-life of 6 hours, which is one of the reasons it is preferred over somatostatin, which has a very short half-life. It is taken up in various neoplastic and inflammatory conditions, as well as by several normal organs:

Tumours
- Paraganglioma, including phaeochromocytoma, although MIBG is preferred for this tumour because of renal accumulation of octreotide
- Pituitary adenoma: if a growth hormone-secreting tumour is 'hot' on a labelled octreotide study, it is likely that the tumour will respond to regular octreotide therapy
- Islet cell tumours, but note that about 40% of insulinomas are negative
- Adrenal neuroblastoma
- Pulmonary small cell tumours: 80% have somatostatin receptors
- Lymphoma
- Medullary thyroid cancer
- Carcinoid (of GI and chest origin)
- Breast cancer
- Meningiomas/astrocytomas

Sarcoidosis

Autoimmune diseases
- Grave's disease
- Rheumatoid joints

Normal organs
- Kidneys and bladder
- Liver and spleen
- Pituitary
- Lung (after radiotherapy or bleomycin)

Operation sites

40 a) **False** Focal nodular hyperplasia is one of only a few focal liver lesions with sufficient Kupffer cells to cause normal or increased uptake of sulphur colloid. Appearances vary and depend on lesion size, but about 10% are 'hot', 60% 'normal' and 40% 'cold'. Other 'hot' liver lesions on sulphur colloid scans include a regenerating nodule and the caudate lobe in Budd–Chiari/inferior vena cava obstruction.

b) **True** ^{99m}Tc pertechnetate (or DTPA) scanning is very sensitive to the presence of testicular torsion, although it has been largely replaced by more widely available ultrasound. Signs of torsion include: a testis with less activity than the opposite testis or adjacent thigh; the 'nubbin' sign, which is increased activity from the iliac artery to just above the testicle secondary to increased flow in the pudendal artery; the 'ring' or 'bull's eye' sign, which is peripheral activity in an inflamed dartos muscle (supplied by the pudendal vessels) with a central photopenic testicle. Scintigraphy cannot diagnose torsion in very small testes, such as in boys under 2 years of age, or in the testicular appendages.

c) **False** Lymphoscintigraphy involves subcutaneous injection of ^{99m}Tc nanocolloid into web space, followed by dynamic scans as the tracer ascends the lymphatic system. It is often performed to diagnose suspected congenital lymphoedema (Milroy's disease), when tracer is seen to pool in the foot. Conversely, increased lymphatic drainage may be seen in venous oedema. It cannot reliably be used to identify malignant involvement of nodes as the resolution is inadequate, but it can be used to guide surgery by identifying the sentinel node.

d) **False** Cisternography involves injection of ^{111}In DTPA or ^{99m}Tc DTPA into the lumbar subarachnoid space and delayed imaging as the tracer moves up the spine into the basal cisterns (seen after 2–4 hours) and over the cerebral hemispheres Oto the vertex (seen after 24–48 hours). Normally, there is no or minimal reflux into the lateral ventricles; transient reflux at 12–24 hours is not significant.

e) **False** In normal pressure hydrocephalus, there is persistent tracer reflux from the basal cisterns into the lateral ventricles, with decreased activity over convexities. There is no ventricular reflux in obstructive hydrocephalus and flow up to convexities is slowed.

Abbreviations

AAA	abdominal aortic aneurysm
ABER	abduction and external rotation
ACA	anterior cerebral artery
ACE	angiotensin-converting enzyme
ACTH	adrenocorticotrophic hormone
ADH	antidiuretic hormone
AML	acute myelolymphoblastic leukaemia
ASD	atrial septal defect
AVM	arteriovenous malformation
BOOP	bronchiolitis obliterans organising pneumonia
BPH	benign prostatic hypertrophy
Bq	becquerel
CAM	cystic adenomatoid malformation
CCK	cholecystokinin
CMV	cytomegalovirus
CNS	central nervous system
COAD	chronic obstructive airway disease
COP	cryptogenic organising pneumonia
COPD	chronic obstructive pulmonary disease
CPA	cerebellopontine angle
CRL	crown-to-rump length
CSF	cerebrospinal fluid
CSP	cavum septi pellucidi
CT	computed tomography
CVA	cerebrovascular accident
DCG	dacryocystography
DCIS	ductal carcinoma *in situ*
DIC	disseminated intravascular coagulation
DIP	desquamative interstitial pneumonia
DISI	dorsal intercalated segmental instability
DMSA	dimercaptosuccinic acid
DSG	dacryoscintigraphy
DTPA	diethylenetriaminepenta-acetic acid
ECA	external cerebral artery/external carotid artery
ESR	erythrocyte sedimentation rate
EUS	endoscopic ultrasonography/ultrasound
FDG	2-[^{18}F]-fluoro-2-deoxy-D-glucose
FMD	fibromuscular dysplasia
FNA	fine-needle aspiration
FNH	focal nodular hyperplasia
GA	gestational age
Ga	gallium
Gd-DTPA	gadopentetate diethylenetriaminepenta-acetic acid
GFR	glomerular filtration rate
GH	growth hormone
GI	gastrointestinal
HCG	human chorionic gonadotrophin
HIDA	hepato-iminodiacetic acid
HIVE	HIV encephalopathy
HMPAO	hexamethylpropyleneamineoxime

HRCT	high resolution computed tomography
HSE	herpes simplex encephalitis
HSV	herpes simplex virus
HU	Hounsfield units
I	iodine
ICA	internal carotid artery
IDA	iminodiacetic acid
IMA	inferior mesenteric artery
In	indium
IVC	inferior vena cava
LDH	lactate dehydrogenase
LVEF	left ventricular ejection fraction
MAA	macroaggregated albumin
MAG_3	mercaptoacetyltriglycine
MALT	mucosal-associated lymphoid tissue
MBq	megabecquerel
MCA	middle cerebral artery
MDP	methylene diphosphonate
MEN	multiple endocrine neoplasia
MIBG	metaiodobenzylguanidine
MIBI	methoxyisobutylisonitrile
MO	molybdenum
MRCP	magnetic resonance cholangiopancreatography
MRI	magnetic resonance imaging
NF	neurofibromatosis
NF-1	neurofibromatosis type 1
NF-2	neurofibromatosis type 2
NHL	non-Hodgkin's lymphoma
NPH	normal pressure hydrocephalus
PAVM	pulmonary arteriovenous malformation
PDA	patent ductus arteriosus
PET	positron emission tomography
PHPV	persistent hyperplastic primary vitreous
PIOPED	Prospective Investigation of Pulmonary Embolism Diagnosis
PML	progressive multifocal encephalopathy
PMMA	polymethylmethacrylate
PNET	primitive neuroectodermal tumours
PPS	parapharyngeal space
PSA	prostate-specific antigen
PTC	percutaneous transhepatic cholangiography
PTFE	polytetrafluoroethylene
PTH	parathyroid hormone
RAS	renal artery stenosis
RB-ILD	respiratory bronchiolitis-interstitial lung disease
RI	resistive index
RIF	right iliac fossa
ROI	region of interest
SAH	subarachnoid haemorrhage
SLAP	superior labral anterior-posterior
SLE	systemic lupus erythematosus

SMA	superior mesenteric artery
SONK	spontaneous osteonecrosis of the knee
SPECT	single photon emission computed tomography
SUV	standardised uptake value
SVC	superior vena cava
SVCO	superior vena cava obstruction
$t_{1/2}$	half-life
TAPVD	total anomalous pulmonary venous drainage
TB	tuberculosis
t_{biol}	biological half-life
Tc	technecium
t_{eff}	effective half-life
TGA	transposition of the great arteries
Tl	thallium
THR	total hip replacement
TIPS	transjugular intrahepatic porto-systemic shunts
tPA	tissue plasminogen activator
TPN	total parenteral nutrition
t_{phys}	physical half-life
TRUS	transrectal ultrasound
UAE	uterine artery embolisation
UIP	usual interstitial pneumonitis
VHL	von Hippel–Lindau syndrome
VISI	ventral intercalated segmental instability
V/Q	ventilation/perfusion
VSD	ventricular septal defects

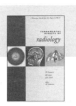

PART 2B FRCR RAPID REPORTING SELF ASSESSMENT CD-ROM

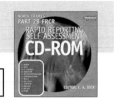

Editor
Elizabeth Dick (UK)

Compiled by radiology registrars, the Part 2B FRCR Rapid Reporting Self Assessment CD-ROM features 10 packets of rapid reporting films; each containing 30 single films that range in difficulty. In view of the changed format of the Part 2B FRCR examination, this CD-ROM provides candidates with an invaluable revision aid and offers useful strategic advice for approaching rapid reporting. Although this resource is primarily aimed at those currently working towards Part 2B of the FRCR it is also suitable for any trainee radiologist or A&E radiographer who reports films in 'hot-seat' sessions or on-call.

"Interactive computer-based education is all too often a demonstration of technical wizardry with little educational value. This CD is a true exception. Computer technology has enabled 300 films to be presented in a quiz format that almost precisely mimics the examination itself."

Prof Peter Armstrong, President of the Royal College of Radiologists

Contents:
10 packets of 30 single films

Available NOW from bmjbookshop.com

March 2000

CD-ROM Microsoft Windows and Apple Macintosh compatible

ISBN: 1 901346 13 7

US$40 / £25 / €40 (plus VAT)

EMERGENCY RADIOLOGY
Rules and tools

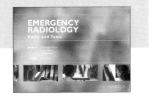

Editor
Jane Young: Whittington Hospital, UK

Authors
Elizabeth Dick: St Mary's Hospital, UK; Ian Francis: The Royal Free Hospital, UK;
Ian Renfrew: Middlesex Hospital, UK

Emergency Radiology stands out from other Accident & Emergency books. No other book specifically targets those new to reporting or reviewing emergency X-rays or those finding themselves in 'hot seat' reporting situations.

The book contains 100 case studies, enabling readers to test themselves on both common and rare and easy-to-miss fractures. The book is divided anatomically. Each chapter begins by setting out the 'rules and tools' on approaching suspected fractures in each anatomical region, before moving on to the case studies. Particular attention has been paid to fractures that are rarely seen, but are vital to spot, such as cervical spine injuries. In addition, normal films are included to mimic the reality of emergency film reporting. Clear X-rays and concise practical answers ensure that this book can be consulted in everyday situations.

"...I wish this book had been available to me at the start of my first job in A&E. It is about as comprehensive as a small book on a massive subject can be. The case studies comprise stories which sound all too familiar to a battle-worn emergency physician!"

Jonathan Wyatt, The Royal Cornwall Hospital

Contents:
• Skull & face
• Spine & axial skeleton
• Upper limb
• Lower limb
• General radiology films
• Normal films

Available NOW from bmjbookshop.com, amazon.com and amazon.co.uk

April 2003

300pp

ISBN: 1 901346 28 5

US$40 / £25 / €40

INTERVENTIONAL RADIOLOGY

Authors

Ian Francis (UK) & Anthony Watkinson (UK)

The growth of real time imaging and technological advances in the design of guide wires, catheters and balloons have seen interventional radiology evolve rapidly over the last 30 years. Such is the pace of these developments that it is difficult to keep up-to-date with changes in this sub-specialty of radiology. This book provides clear information on the indications, techniques, and outcomes of the full spectrum of interventional procedures, in a format that will appeal to general radiologists, clinicians, and general practitioners alike.

"This book is nicely produced with clear images and the authors are to be congratulated on condensing so much information into such a concise and accessible format... There are sections covering all aspects of radiological intervention and the descriptions of the techniques and their application is very much up to date."

Irving Wells, *Clinical Radiology*

Contents:
- General interventional radiology
- Gastrointestinal intervention
- Hepatobiliary intervention
- Uroradiological intervention
- Vascular intervention
- Gynecological intervention

Available NOW from bmjbookshop.com, amazon.com and amazon.co.uk

January 2001

165pp

ISBN: 1 901346 02 1

ISSN: 1472-4138

US$30 / £20 / €30

IMAGING IN STROKE

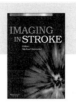

Editor
Michael Hennerici: University of Heidelberg, Mannheim, Germany

Authors
Julien Bogousslavsky (Switzerland), Gabriel De Freitas (Brazil), Wolf-Dieter Heiss (Germany), Olav Jansen (Germany), Christoph Koch (Germany), Thomas Kucinski (Germany), Joachim Liepert (Germany), Stephen Meairs (Germany), Michael Moseley (Usa), Tobias Neumann-Haefelin (Germany), Fabienne Perren (Switzerland), Cornelius Weiller (Germany), Hermann Zeumer (Germany)

Neuroimaging techniques are crucial in the management of stroke patients. This book is an important resource in the quest to better understand stroke and its heterogeneity. After a first chapter on the classification of stroke, it outlines that the neuroimaging techniques are not only useful to diagnose stroke, its mechanisms and its causes, but is also an important tool to improve our knowledge on the pathophysiology of stroke and of its recovery. This book has involved prestigious contributors who have a great knowledge on this topic, and are skilled at describing the current state of knowledge, and also at projecting developments that are likely to occur in the future. This book is useful for all those who have to manage stroke patients at the acute stage, or later, i.e. neurologists, stroke specialists, rehabilitation physicians, and neuroradiologists, and finally for all those who are in search of a focused authoritative review on this subject. It will assume a prominent place as a reference.

"Professor Hennerici and his colleagues provide a clear, beautifully written, cutting edge, and comprehensive overview on what neuroimaging techniques may provide in terms of diagnostic tools and understanding of the pathophysiology of stroke and of its recovery. Its content is of major interest for an optimal management of stroke patients, which requires a sound understanding and an accurate diagnosis."

Didier Leys, University of Lille, France

Contents:
- Introduction
- Classification of stroke
- CT in acute stroke
- MRI in acute stroke
- CTA and MRA in stroke
- Neurosonology in acute stroke
- Intracerebral hemorrhage
- Applications of positron emission tomography in ischemic stroke
- Recovery and plasticity imaging in stroke patients

Available NOW from bmjbookshop.com, amazon.com and amazon.co.uk

April 2003

216pp

ISBN: 1 901346 25 0

US$45 / £30 / €45

BRAIN IMAGING IN EPILEPSY

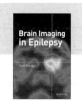

Author
David D Maudgil: The Royal Free Hospital, UK

Recent advances in functional neuroimaging have greatly enhanced our ability to visualize and develop a greater understanding of brain processes at work. This book provides an overview of the techniques that have been developed, including positron emission tomography, single photon emission computed tomography, functional magnetic resonance imaging, diffusion weighted imaging, and magnetic resonance spectroscopy. Relevant features of the basic neuroscience of epilepsy are reviewed and the application of these techniques in diagnosing, treating and developing new treatments for epilepsy is discussed.

"In this excellent monograph, Dr Maudgil has done all of us a service in highlighting the possibilities for imaging and subsequent treatment in this too-often ignored disease. I believe if this work is read by all neurologists and radiologists who come into contact with patients suffering epilepsy, their minds will be opened to a new and fascinating world."

John Buscombe, Consultant Nuclear Medicine Physician, Royal Free Hospital, London, UK

Contents:
• Epilepsy
• Imaging techniques for epilepsy
• Characteristic clinical and EEG findings in epilepsy syndromes
• Clinical applications of functional imaging
• Future developments

Available NOW from bmjbookshop.com, amazon.com and amazon.co.uk

August 2003

110pp

ISBN: 1 901346 24 2

US$24 / £15 / €24